The Master Boxer

The Definitive Guide to Becoming a
World Class Fighter

Bryant Perrella
"Goodfella"

The Master Boxer:
The Definitive Guide to Becoming a World Class Fighter

By Bryant "Goodfella" Perrella

- Hardcover ISBN: 979-8-9929773-0-1
- Paperback ISBN: 979-8-9929773-2-5
- eBook ISBN: 979-8-9929773-1-8

Cover Design: Julian Munoz
Interior Formatting & Illustrations: Ana Simmons
Developmental Editing: Christine Bucher
Copy Editing: Harri Aston

First Edition September 2025
Written April 2023-March 2025

For information about permission to reproduce selections from this book, write to: info@bryantperrella.com

Official Website: bryantperrella.com
Instagram, Facebook, X: @bryantperrella

Published by Bryant Goodfella Perrella LLC

Printed in the United States of America

Acknowledgements

Boxing has been the ultimate test. A journey filled with triumphs, setbacks and sacrifices. It has shaped me in ways nothing else could, demanding everything physically, mentally and financially. But through all the ups and downs, I've never walked this path alone.

To my coaches: each of you played a role in shaping me into the fighter I became.

John Doherty (RIP), for being the first to see my potential and instilling the belief in me to pursue this sport. If it weren't for him, I wouldn't have continued.

Steven J. Canton, owner of SJC Boxing, for opening your doors to me. The first boxing gym I ever stepped foot into, setting everything in motion.

Larry Willis, for being a major part of my amateur years and helping guide my transition into the pros. When I first walked into your gym, I knew this is where I needed to be. You instilled in me the importance of speed. Fast hands, sharp combinations, and letting my hands fly!

Jose Ojeda, for always being there when I needed you. Solid, dependable, and a big part of shaping my career from the amateur days on.

Joel Pagan, from the first day you saw me, you believed you saw greatness. We trained hard. You covered everything: boxing, mindset, nutrition, strength and conditioning. Your positive affirmations always went a long way.

Michael Nowling, we achieved a lot together. We made it to the big stage, through the highest highs and the lowest lows. You were a huge help through it all and always made sure I had what I needed. We did so much with so little for so long, we learned how to make something out of nothing. I'm grateful for everything we accomplished during our time.

Kelvin Torres, my boy who got me war ready for many fights. We put in overtime, all the time! You weren't just my S&C coach, you were in the trenches with me. From brutal circuits to late-night boxing sessions, you pushed me past my limits and sharpened every weapon. You played a huge role in helping turn me into a beast, and you showed me just how far we could push the limits in training. You were also a key part of me getting signed by Al Haymon, and I never forgot that.

Carlos Vargas, my cutman. Thanks for being in my corner, always ready to handle any cuts that might have come my way. Your readiness and presence gave me confidence every time I stepped into the ring.

Travis Bonyfield, thanks for helping me with my strength and conditioning for an important fight. We came out with a dominant win. Appreciate you being part of that camp.

To the trainers at IronDNA Fitness, for helping me power-up for some big fights. The work we put in together added another layer to my preparation, and it made a real difference when everything was on the line.

Jesse Reid, the bridge to recognizing the higher levels of knowledge and experience that were out there. You also stepped in the corner for some big fights, and it gave me confidence in having that kind of wisdom in my corner when it counted.

Roy Jones Jr., for revealing the deeper layers of boxing: the real chess game, and expanding my understanding of technique and strategy beyond anything I had known before. You had the patience and persistence to keep drilling and correcting my mistakes, and that played a big role in making me a much more intelligent, capable fighter.

Sebastian Lopez, for being a huge asset in preparing me for my junior middleweight debut. Your analytical mind, combat sports expertise, and focus on physical preparation made a real difference when it mattered most.

Billy Lyell, former world middleweight title contender and owner of Sweet Science Boxing & Fitness, for being a great friend, supporter and coach who played a role in my development. You're big on mindset, and with your experience as a former pro boxer, you brought insight that was truly invaluable.

Joe Rojas, for all the work on the mitts and the time spent sharpening my skills. The work we put in made a difference, and that never went unnoticed.

Sergei Belovolov, for introducing me to the Russian power boxing style and always pushing my limits. You're a great person and a great teacher. Even with the language barrier, we made it work. Because in that sense, boxing is a universal language.

Tony Morgan, for drilling it into me to keep my damn head back and teaching me how to use my reach more effectively.

Michel Sarduy, for helping enhance my footwork with some Cuban style and for playing a key role in my preparation for a big fight.

Sam Payne, for putting me through the ringer in camp for an amateur tournament and showing me another style that could be used. 'Pressure breaks pipes' — and you made sure I understood that.

Jeff Knorr, always willing to help however needed. Whether it was holding mitts, offering advice, or just being there during preparation. More than anything, I'm grateful for the support and your friendship through it all.

Pat Wilson, for helping me through some tough weight cuts for big fights and being a strong support when it counted most. Thank you for everything you did behind the scenes.

Todd Harlib (RIP), for helping connect the dots and opening doors that pushed my career forward. Your support came through when it mattered, and I'll always value that.

Keith Thurman and Dan Birmingham, for creating pivotal stages in my career and believing in me when it counted. It meant a lot, and I'm thankful for the experience and everything that came with it.

To the promoters I've worked with along the way, thank you for believing in me and giving me the opportunity to showcase my talent. None of this would have been possible without you. A special thanks to Al Haymon and Premier Boxing Champions, it's been a pleasure working with you. And to TGB Promotions, thank you for being part of my path and for the opportunities to compete on major stages.

To my sponsors and those who stood by me when times were tough. You didn't just believe in my career; you believed in me.

A special thanks to Michael Farrar, the businessman who owns Whelco and ACT (Automation & Control Technologies), as well as Fitness 4 All Boxercise. A sponsor, but above all, a dear friend. You are always looking for ways to push me forward. Whether through support, connections, or simply being there when it counted. I truly appreciate everything you've done for me along the way.

To my father, Al, my mother, Melissa, and my Oma. Your support, whether in life, in boxing, or in shaping my relationship with reading, has played a role in my journey.

And to someone who has been instrumental, not only in the making of this book, but in many corners of my life and career. You know who you are. Your impact has been invaluable, and my real secret weapon.

Boxing has been more than a sport; it's been my life, my passion, my greatest teacher. The fire that it lit in me will never fade, and everything it has given me continues to drive me forward.

Thank You All.

Table of Contents

Round 4: Training Blueprint

Round 5: Physical Development

Round 6: Endurance & Conditioning

Round 7: Recovery & Nutrition

Round 8: Your Team

Before the First Bell

I wasn't supposed to be writing this. I was supposed to be training.

Instead, I'm here with a swollen hand. Another surgery. Another fork in the road.

They don't tell you what happens when the crowd stops.

When the adrenaline fades and you're staring at your own fist, wondering if you'll ever throw it again.

For the first time, I had to ask myself: Am I done?

I've given most of my life to this game.

Not just the fights, the hours alone in the gym, the studying, and the mistakes that shaped my understanding more than any win ever did.

If this is the last time I speak as a fighter...

Then this book is the transmission I leave behind.

It's not motivational. It's not theory.

It's the truth—the kind you only find when your body fails, but your understanding deepens.

If I make it back to the ring... good.

If I don't... this book is the return, and the introduction of something much bigger.

Introduction: The Way of the Ring

Boxing goes far beyond being a sport. It's a test of mind, body, and heart. From the outside, it might look like two fighters in a ring, throwing punches at each other, aiming to win. But anyone who's stepped between those ropes knows it's so much more. Boxing demands discipline, strategy, resilience, and sacrifice. Every jab. Every feint. Every counterpunch. They're built on countless hours of training, mental conditioning, and hard-earned experience. That's what it takes to strive toward becoming a world-class fighter.

I've lived this journey. After years as a professional boxer, with wins, losses, injuries *(including working through hand surgery as I write this book),* and countless rounds of preparation, I've learned that success in the ring is about far more than brute strength or flashy techniques.

Boxing is like high-speed chess: it's about thinking two steps ahead, reading your opponent, and making quick, calculated decisions under pressure. But it's also extremely physical, demanding peak conditioning, sharp reflexes and raw endurance. The mental and physical sides of the sport are deeply connected.

When I first started learning this sport, it was through a "how to box" book from the local library. Now, after years in the ring, and with the uncertainty of my return, it feels only right to give back in the same way: by passing on the experience and lessons I've gained throughout my journey.

The Master Boxer is the guide I wish I had when I first laced up my gloves. It brings together the lessons I've learned from years of fighting, training, research, and trial and error, alongside perspectives from mentors and studying the greats. This book is the culmination of many things I've absorbed: carefully crafted and organized to provide you with high-level insights, techniques and strategies that will elevate your boxing game.

In these pages, you'll find valuable knowledge in key areas: fitness routines to build explosive power and endurance, recovery techniques to keep your body strong, and the mindset needed to handle pressure. You'll also learn boxing strategies, including how to fight against different styles and properly peak for fight night, all of which will give you a significant edge over your opponent.

From weight-cutting methods to preparing you mentally and physically, and much more, this book offers practical advice you can tailor to your own journey, giving you the freedom to absorb what's useful and discard what's not. This isn't a book you read once and put away. It's a guide meant to grow with you. Something you can return to again and again, picking out the principles and tactics that best serve you at different stages of your training and career.

Truthfully, boxing isn't just about who hits harder; it's about who thinks faster, moves smarter, and stays focused when the pressure is on. This book acts as your corner coach, offering real-world strategies to help you sharpen your skills and perform at your best. It's more than a guide or blueprint, it includes exercises, drills and training ideas you can experiment with to see what works best for you. My aim is simple: to provide value through the wisdom I've gathered, helping you navigate the sport with confidence and clarity.

Whether you're new to boxing or an experienced fighter looking to sharpen your skills, this guide is designed to help you reach new heights. Becoming a better boxer isn't about talent alone, it's about preparation, strategy, and relentless dedication to improving every part of your game.

Inside, you'll find the tools that can transform you from a beginner into a fighter with the potential to reach world-class levels. The ring may be unforgiving, but with the right preparation and understanding, it's also where you claim your throne of greatness.

Lessons That Forge a Fighter

Before the bell rings, a boxer stands alone, thinking about the discipline, focus, and hard work that led to this moment. Boxing is a place where you learn some of life's biggest lessons. Inside the ring, in what boxing pundits sometimes call the squared circle, every challenge faced and every victory earned shows the strength and determination that make a champion. But these lessons don't stay in the ring; they carry over into every part of life. Boxing shapes more than your body. It carves out your character. The discipline built during training, the focus honed in the ring, and the perseverance shown in every fight become a part of who you are. These qualities go beyond the gym and ring, helping you face life's challenges with the same determination. Whether it's a tough day at work or a personal setback, the toughness you've developed through boxing will help you push through.

As you start your journey in boxing, remember that the lessons you learn here will serve you both inside and outside the ring. Treat every training session, every sparring match, and every fight as a chance to grow. Not merely as a fighter, but as a person.

Round 1: Fundamentals & Technique

Chapter 1
The Allure of the Sweet Science

In the dim glow of the gym lights, the rhythmic beat of the speed bag echoes as a young fighter laces up his gloves, ready to step into a journey taken by countless legends before him. Boxing, known as the "Sweet Science", pulls people in with its perfect mix of strategy, strength and stamina. It's a sport that demands everything but rewards you with unmatched returns, both physically and mentally. In this chapter, we'll explore the deep history of boxing, the transformative power it holds, and the timeless appeal that keeps luring fighters into the ring.

The Storied Past of Pugilism

Boxing has ancient roots, dating back to pre-Roman Greece, where it was a celebrated sport in the original Olympic Games. Both warriors and gladiators participated in these pugilistic contests, demonstrating their strength and skill.

Modern boxing began to take shape in 18th and 19th century England. Originally a bare-knuckle sport associated with gambling and underground events, it evolved with the introduction of the Marquess of Queensberry rules in the 1800s. These rules, which required gloves, set time limits, and banned dangerous tactics, transformed boxing into a legitimate and widely respected sport.

The Body and Mind in Harmony

Boxing is more than physical strength. It's a mix of power, speed and sharp mental focus. The health benefits are profound. High-intensity boxing workouts can burn between 500 and 800 calories per hour, depending on your weight and intensity, according to estimates based on metabolic studies and fitness research[1]. The constant movement improves cardiovascular

---

[1] Calorie burn estimates based on metabolic equivalent (MET) research for high-intensity boxing activities including heavy bag work and sparring. BleGend Gym fitness analysis, 2023.

health and builds strength and endurance, especially in the arms, shoulders and core.

The benefits go beyond physical health. The focus, concentration and quick reflexes required in boxing sharpen your mind and hand-eye coordination. As renowned boxing coach Freddie Roach says: *"Boxing trains your brain as much as your body."* It's also an excellent stress reliever, offering a way to release built-up energy and frustration. Many people find that the rhythmic movement, combined with the intense focus required for throwing punches, creating movement patterns and executing footwork, not only has a meditative effect that clears the mind but also serves as a powerful outlet for built-up tension. Most importantly, learning boxing builds strong self-confidence. As you overcome challenges like grueling training sessions, mental hurdles and tough opponents, you'll feel a sense of accomplishment that positively impacts all areas of your life.

The Journey of Becoming a Boxer

Whether you dream of becoming a professional or just want to improve your fitness and learn self-defense, boxing offers something for everyone. The atmosphere at a boxing gym is welcoming, bringing together people from all walks of life who share a love for the sport. It's a supportive environment that fosters camaraderie, motivation and personal growth.

Boxing is more than a sport. It's a lifestyle. It teaches discipline, resilience and perseverance. It challenges you to face your fears, push past your limits, and discover your true potential. With its rich history, deep traditions and the unbreakable human spirit, boxing offers physical and mental challenges that can shape your life.

Take that first step. Put on your gloves, step into the ring, and embrace the art of boxing. As Muhammad Ali said: "Even the greatest was once a beginner." Your journey to greatness starts now.

Chapter 2
The Importance of Fundamentals

"There are no masters of ANY craft who haven't mastered the fundamentals first! It's a rite of passage required before you can truly take things to the next level." [2]
—Lennox Lewis, legendary heavyweight champion

Boxing, like any skill-based sport, is built on a foundation of essential techniques. These basics may seem simple, but they're the core of all advanced skills. Whether you're new to the ring or have years of experience, honing these key elements is vital to your success as a fighter.

Why Fundamentals Matter

No matter where you are in your boxing journey, the fundamentals remain central. They tie together every stage of development, from beginner to advanced. These basics prepare you for more complex techniques, they guarantee that when you use them, you do so with accuracy, power and effectiveness.

The path to boxing greatness starts with a strong foundation, and it's up to you to build it, one brick at a time.

Building a Strong Foundation

Just like a house needs a solid base, a boxer needs strong fundamentals to succeed. Skills like stance, punching form, footwork and defense are crucial. Without them, you'll never reach your full potential. Strong core techniques also help you maintain balance and control, making your movements precise and allowing your punches to land with maximum power.

Boosting Punch Effectiveness

Proper technique makes every punch more effective, whether you're focusing on power, speed or precision. Perfecting the

---

[2] Lewis, Lennox. X (formerly Twitter) post, @LennoxLewis, January 24, 2018.

basics allows you to adapt to different situations in the ring, making sure each strike is delivered with intent and impact.

Refinement Through Repetition

"Repetition is the mother of memory."[3] Boxing requires dedication, perseverance and a willingness to repeat these movements until they become second nature. As you advance, revisiting these core skills will keep you sharp. Over time, what once felt basic will evolve with your growing strength, accuracy and expertise.

Tip: Keep a training journal to track your progress and reflect on your improvements.

Success in the ring comes not from perfection but from relentless progress. Each punch, each move, each round is a chance to grow stronger and more skilled.

A Note for Advanced Boxers

If you're confident in your fundamentals, you may be ready to dive deeper into advanced strategies and concepts in later chapters. This book covers important topics like strategy, setups, fight preparation, mindset, physical conditioning and nutrition, key components for unlocking your full potential in the ring. But no matter how advanced you get, revisiting the basics will always keep your foundation strong and your skills dangerous.

---

[3] "Repetitio mater memoriae" (Latin proverb).

Chapter 3
The Fighter's Arsenal:
Punch Like a Pro

"Practice doesn't make perfect. Perfect practice makes perfect." [4]
—Vince Lombardi, legendary NFL coach

Boxing requires a unique combination of skill, strategy and discipline. Before stepping into the ring, it's important to develop these necessary techniques by building on the basics. In this chapter, we'll cover the fundamentals every aspiring boxer must develop on their path to greatness, along with the main punches that form the core of your offensive arsenal.

The Boxing Stance

Your stance, how you position your body to fight, is the bedrock upon which all other techniques are built. A proper boxing stance is all about balance, comfort and efficiency. It's generally recommended to fight from a stance that matches your dominant hand, as it positions your strongest punches in the rear, giving them more power. However, not all fighters stick to this rule. Some adopt a stance that feels more natural or offers strategic advantages. For instance, Oscar De La Hoya, a natural left-hander, fought from an orthodox stance, using his lead hand for powerful hooks and uppercuts. Similarly, Winky Wright, a right-hander, found success with a southpaw stance, crafting one of the best jabs in boxing.

It's worth experimenting with both the orthodox and southpaw stances to see what feels best for you. Trying both sides can help you discover hidden strengths. Over time, you may even develop both, leading to better versatility and ambidexterity, which will keep your opponents off balance and make it harder to anticipate your moves. Ultimately, the choice is individual and

---

[4] Lombardi, Vince. Quote attributed to legendary NFL coach and motivational speaker. Often cited in coaching and sports psychology contexts.

depends on your personal goals and style, which can evolve over time.

Orthodox Stance

What it is: The most common stance for right-handed fighters. In the orthodox stance, your left foot is forward, and your left hand is the lead hand for jabs, while your stronger right hand stays back to throw power punches like crosses and hooks.

Feet Positioning: Position your left foot forward, with your right foot turned inward slightly, roughly shoulder-width apart or a bit wider.

Hand Positioning: Your left hand is the lead guard, staying high to protect your face, while your right hand stays at the rear, ready to launch powerful punches.

Southpaw Stance

What it is: The stance used by left-handed fighters. In the southpaw stance, the right foot is forward, and the right hand is the lead hand for jabs, while the left hand stays back, delivering strong power punches.

Feet Positioning: Position your right foot forward, with your left foot behind, slightly turned inward, at a width that allows for stability and quick movement.

Hand Positioning: Your right hand becomes the lead guard, and the left hand stays poised at the rear to unleash power shots.

Body Positioning

Feet Placement

For both orthodox and southpaw stances, foot placement should allow for both stability and mobility. Most fighters stand with their feet slightly wider than shoulder-width, but this varies based on individual style and movement preferences. A wider stance can provide more balance and power for some fighters but may reduce mobility, while a narrower stance allows for quicker movement but can affect stability. Your ideal stance depends on your fighting style, reach, and comfort in the ring.

Knee Bend

Bend your knees slightly, distributing your weight evenly between both feet. This keeps you fluid and ready to shift, punch or defend from any angle without sacrificing control.

Knuckle Position

The way you position your knuckles on impact can vary depending on what feels natural and effective for you. For example, many boxers prefer to land a hook with their thumb pointing upwards, keeping the fist in a more vertical position. Others prefer to turn the wrist over slightly, landing with the knuckles more horizontal. Similarly, using a vertical fist position during an uppercut might feel more comfortable in certain situations. Both approaches are valid, and it's about finding what feels right for you and fits the situation. However, it is generally advised to aim to make contact with the first two knuckles to ensure proper alignment and reduce the risk of injury.

Common Mistakes

Leaning too far forward, overextending the rear hand, or improper foot placement can throw you off balance and open you up to counters. Focus on maintaining good posture, evenly distributing your weight, keeping a strong base and staying light on your feet to remain mobile.

One of the best ways to recognize these issues is through self-awareness and feedback. Checking a mirror while shadow boxing can help you spot posture and balance mistakes in real time. Recording your training sessions allows you to review your movement and catch details you might miss in the moment. Having a coach or trainer analyze your positioning is invaluable, as they can correct subtle errors before they become habits. Additionally, sparring partners can give immediate feedback, if they're consistently able to counter you after certain movements, it's a sign something needs adjusting.

> **Tip:** Finding the perfect stance takes time, but it's worth the effort. Try different variations and adjust your stance to suit your natural movement and balance.

Drill

Practice shadow boxing in front of a mirror to correct your form and balance. Use each session to adjust and perfect your stance, whether you're in orthodox or southpaw.

The Power of the Punch

> *"Sure the fight was fixed. I fixed it with a right hand."* [5]—George Foreman, legendary heavyweight champion

Punching is the heart and soul of boxing. From quick jabs to devastating hooks and uppercuts, each punch serves a specific purpose. But more than just technique, it's how you engage your entire body that creates real power in your punches.

Key Elements of a Powerful Punch

Use Your Body: Rotate your hips and shoulders as you extend your arm. This rotation generates power from your core and legs, not just your arm.

Stay Relaxed: Tension in your shoulders, arms or hands can slow down your punches and drain your energy. Keep your body loose and fluid, allowing your movements to flow naturally. Relaxation also helps you generate speed and snap, making your punches more effective. If you find yourself tightening up, focus on controlled breathing—take slow, deep breaths between exchanges to reset your composure. Keep your hands relaxed when not punching to avoid unnecessary tension in your arms

---

[5] Foreman, George. Speaking after he knocked out Michael Moorer to become a world heavyweight champion again, aged 45, on November 5, 1994.

and shoulders. Between exchanges, lightly bounce your shoulders to release tightness. Subtle movements, like shifting your weight or bouncing on your toes, can also prevent stiffness and help maintain fluidity in your movements.

Weight Transfer: As your punch connects, transfer your weight with it, towards the target to ensure your striking blow has maximum force behind it.

Protect While You Attack: When throwing punches, especially power punches, avoid dropping your opposite hand. Keep it tight against your temple, as if holding a phone to your ear. Dropping your guard can leave you vulnerable to counters while delivering your own strike.

Keep Elbows Close: Keep your elbows close to your body to avoid flaring your arms out. This helps maintain proper form so the power comes from the rotation of your body rather than arm strength alone.

Punch Through the Target: Focus on punching through the target, not just at it. This mindset helps you drive your punch deeper and deliver more impact. Aim two to three inches behind the head when throwing knockout blows.

Energy Efficiency and Relaxation

Relaxation is one of the most overlooked weapons in boxing, but it's a major key to energy efficiency and endurance. Staying relaxed as you throw punches prevents unnecessary tension in your shoulders, arms and body, which can quickly drain your stamina. Proper breathing plays a critical role here. Exhale sharply as you throw each punch to engage your core and add snap to your strikes.

For most punches, a sharp exhalation at impact creates maximum speed and power. However, in certain situations, such as when throwing short-range body shots or inside hooks, you may find that slightly extending your exhalation and 'sinking' the punch into the target can help transfer more force. This can be especially useful for body shots, where deeper force absorption can wear an opponent down over time rather than just knocking them back. That said, extending contact time also increases the risk of being countered, so it's something to experiment with and apply strategically rather than relying on it for every inside shot.

Inhale during non-engagement moments to replenish oxygen and stay composed. Fighters who tense up or hold their breath while punching burn excess energy, often tiring out sooner than necessary. The ability to stay relaxed has a dramatic effect on how long your stamina lasts in the ring. The more tension you carry, the more energy you waste. This can lead to unnecessary fatigue, even if your conditioning is solid.

Relaxation also helps with the snap of a punch, which I'll cover further in this chapter. By focusing on relaxation, you'll not only throw more fluid punches but also maintain your endurance throughout the fight. It's natural to feel tight and tense at first, but as you implement these tips and gain confidence in the ring, staying relaxed will become easier over time.

Reminder!

The power of your punch comes from your entire body, not just your arm. Engage your core and legs to maximize impact.

Common Mistakes

Throwing Arm Punches: Punches that rely solely on the arm without body rotation can reduce your power. Make sure your punches start from the ground up, using your legs and core.

Flaring Arms: Avoid flaring your arms out. Keep them in and aligned with your body to rotate more naturally.

Drill

Spend at least three to four rounds each session shadowboxing, focusing on perfecting your form for each punch. Use a heavy bag to practice power punches with full body engagement.

The Jab

"A good right hand can take you around the block, a good jab will take you around the world." [6] —Cus D'Amato

The jab—a quick, straight punch thrown with your lead hand—is often called the most important punch in boxing. It's fast and versatile, and can set up almost everything else you do in the ring. A great jab can throw off your opponent's rhythm, measure distance, and create openings for more powerful punches.

Technique

Stance: Start in your boxing stance with your lead foot slightly forward, knees bent, and hands up.

Execution: Push off your back foot as you extend your lead hand straight out. Turn your fist so that your palm faces downward at the point of impact, with your chin tucked behind your shoulder. You can also use an advanced variation with a vertical fist (palm facing sideways) to exploit different angles and find openings through your opponent's guard.

When stepping in with the jab, push off your back foot and take a small step forward with your lead foot, landing at the same time the jab snaps out. Then slide your rear foot forward the same distance, bringing you back into stance. When stepping back with the jab, move your rear foot first, throw the jab as you retreat, then follow by stepping your lead foot back the same distance to maintain your balance and positioning.

For the jab to the body, be sure to drop your level before, or during throwing the shot. Bend your knees, lower your stance, and keep your chin tucked. This makes you defensively responsible while still delivering a quick, effective shot to the midsection. Step in slightly with the jab, and be sure to quickly step back to avoid counters.

---

[6] D'Amato, Cus. (Attributed quote). Legendary boxing trainer and manager, most notably of Mike Tyson, Floyd Patterson and José Torres.

Recoil: The jab should be quick and sharp. Immediately retract your hand back to the starting position to maintain your guard.

Keep Your Guard Up: Always keep your rear hand close to your chin for protection, ready to defend or throw a follow-up punch. When throwing a jab, consider keeping your rear hand in front of your face to block or parry an incoming jab, this is especially useful in orthodox vs. orthodox or southpaw vs. southpaw matchups, where simultaneous jabs are common.

Tip: Don't overlook the jab to the body, it's a highly effective punch that can sap your opponent's energy, stop their forward momentum, and create openings for punches up top. Properly executed, it keeps your opponent guessing and wears them down over the course of the fight.

Advanced Tactics: The Educated Jab

Once you've mastered the mechanics of a proper jab, the next step is to elevate it into an educated weapon. An educated jab is used with purpose, intelligence and adaptability, going beyond a basic, mechanical punch. It's thrown as a strategic tool to control the fight and is tailored to fit different situations, often aiding in the ability to control the fight, create opportunities, or disrupt the opponent's rhythm. It's not only a jab for the sake of throwing one, it's a jab with strategy behind it.

Here's a breakdown of what makes a jab educated:

Varied Speed and Power: An educated jab is not always thrown with full power. Sometimes it's light and probing, other times it's stiff and punishing. The *Stiff Jab* is a forceful jab thrown with authority, used to stop an advancing opponent or establish dominance. Unlike a probing jab, it carries more impact and can deter an opponent from rushing in. Because committing to a stiff jab can leave you briefly exposed to counters, it's important to keep your chin tucked behind your lead shoulder as you throw. This built-in defensive habit helps protect you from unseen shots while still delivering a strong, commanding jab.

Purposeful Placement: An educated jab targets different areas , head, body, chest, or even the opponent's gloves, to set up combinations, create openings, or manipulate their guard. One variation is the *Up-Jab*, which is thrown from a lower angle, slipping under an opponent's guard and making it harder to read. This subtle adjustment can add unpredictability to your offense. The *Body Jab* is another effective variation, targeting the midsection to interrupt breathing, break rhythm, and set up follow-up attacks.

Feints and Deception: Feints are deliberate movements or actions designed to fake an attack and bait a reaction from your opponent. When paired with an educated jab, they can disguise your true intentions, forcing your opponent to react in predictable ways. For example, a quick flick of the jab can make them flinch, leaving them open for your next move. (You'll learn more about feints in a dedicated chapter later.)

Used as a Measuring Stick: It gauges the opponent's distance, timing and reactions, helping you determine how they might respond to future attacks. The *Probe Jab* is a light, exploratory jab used to test your opponent's reactions and gather information, such as whether they parry, slip, freeze, or counter. It keeps them occupied without overcommitting, allowing you to set up stronger punches.

Disruption Tool: An educated jab interferes with the opponent's rhythm, keeps them guessing, and prevents them from establishing their offense. It's used as a defensive measure just as much as an offensive one.

Setting Up Combinations: It opens up opportunities for follow-up punches. For example, a double or triple jab can set up a power shot like a cross or hook.

Maintaining Control: An educated jab establishes ring control. It can keep an opponent at bay, as well as allow you to dictate the pace and range of the fight on your terms.

Adapting to the Opponent: It can adjust based on the opponent's style. For example:

- ○ **Against an aggressive fighter:** A well-placed jab to the body can disrupt forward momentum, and make them think twice about rushing in.
- ○ **Against a defensive fighter:** Use it as a probing jab to draw them out of their shell or create opportunities to attack.

The Cross (Straight Right or Straight Left)

A cross is a straight punch thrown with the rear hand, traveling directly from the guard to the target in a straight line. It's a powerful punch typically following a jab, making it one of the most direct and impactful strikes in boxing. The cross is used to capitalize on openings created by your jab and feints.

Technique

Stance: From your boxing stance, make sure your weight is evenly distributed with knees slightly bent.

Execution: Rotate your hips and shoulders as you extend your rear hand straight toward your target. To maximize rotation and power, *think "pull" rather than "push"—violently pull your opposite shoulder back* to drive full-body rotation with speed and force. This explosive, pulling motion of the opposite shoulder generates the speed and power needed to make the cross truly impactful. (This can be used for all other power punches as well.)

When throwing a committed jab-cross combination with forward momentum, step slightly forward with your lead foot as you jab, then slide your rear foot forward behind it as you throw the cross. This maintains stance integrity while allowing maximum leverage, rotational force, and impact.

Power: The power comes from the rotation of your body. Aim to punch through your target.

Return: Bring your hand back to your guard position, keeping your chin tucked behind your shoulder. Weaving under (in a "U" motion) after throwing the cross can also be beneficial to avoid any incoming counter shots.

The Hook

The hook is a devastating punch, coming around the side, and can be aimed at your opponent's head or body.

Technique

Stance: From your boxing stance, keep your elbows bent and aligned with your body.

Execution: Rotate your hips and slightly turn your opposite shoulder before throwing the hook to generate power and balance. Your arm should form a 90-degree angle as you swing it horizontally toward your target. The punch should travel in a tight arc with your elbow up and in line with your fist.

The cross naturally sets you up to rip the hook with force, your body is already rotated, loaded, and primed to unwind into the hook. Each punch builds on the next, transferring momentum and maximizing impact when thrown in sequence.

Target: Aim for your opponent's chin or body, depending on your strategy. The power comes from your core and lower body.

Return: After the punch lands, quickly bring your hand back to your guard position or roll under. Maintain your balance and be ready to defend or follow up.

The Uppercut

The uppercut is a powerful punch that comes from below, aimed at your opponent's chin or body. It's especially effective up close and can be a fight-ender when timed correctly.

Technique

Stance: Start in your boxing stance, with your knees slightly bent.

Execution: Drop your rear shoulder slightly as you dip your knees, then explode upward with your punch. Your fist should travel vertically. Rotate your hips and shoulders to generate power.

The hook naturally puts you in position to fire an uppercut with force, your weight is already shifting and your torso is primed to drive upward. Used together, the hook and uppercut create brutal close-range combinations that flow with power.

Target: Aim for the chin or solar plexus, depending on the situation.

Return: Quickly reset your stance after the punch, bringing your hand back to your guard position. Keep your chin down and be prepared for a counterattack.

The Overhand

The overhand is a powerful, looping punch that comes over your opponent's guard. It's often used to surprise opponents who are expecting straight punches and is generally thrown with your rear hand. This punch can also be thrown with the lead hand as an advanced variation.

Technique

Stance: Begin in your boxing stance, keeping your weight balanced.

Execution: Drop your rear shoulder slightly and dip your knees as you load up for the punch. Then, bring your rear hand over and down in a looping motion, aiming to come over the top of your opponent's guard.

Target: Aim for your opponent's temple, jaw, or the side of their head. The overhand is particularly effective if your opponent is dropping their hands to block body shots or if their posture is too high and standing upright.

Return: Let your punch continue its natural arc, but be ready to quickly get back to position. The overhand leaves you momentarily exposed, so quick recovery is crucial.

Putting It All Together

Learning basic punches is just the start. Practice them until they become instinctive, and you can throw them cleanly when it matters most. Success in boxing comes from repetition and constant improvement. The more you practice, the more these movements become second nature.

Remember, each punch has its purpose, and understanding when and how to use them is just as important as the technique itself. As you progress in your training, you'll start to see how these punches can be combined and adapted to suit your style and strategy.

Staying Safe in the Danger Zone: Navigating The Centerline

In boxing, the centerline is an imaginary vertical line running down the middle of your body. It represents the path along which straight punches, like jabs and crosses, or powerful overhands are thrown. When you're in your opponent's punching range, what we'll call the danger zone, where the risk of getting tagged increases significantly , it's important to be aware of this line to avoid getting hit. At this distance, you can rely on defensive tools like parrying, slipping, ducking, rolling, or keeping your head further back to avoid punches altogether.

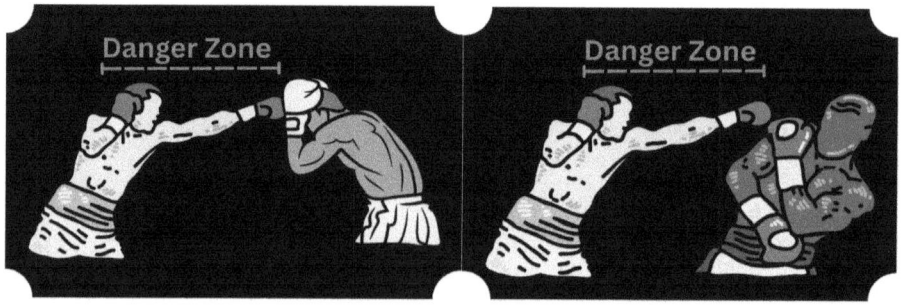

Why Awareness of the Centerline Matters

If you stay on the centerline too long, you're an easy target. Your opponent's punches will travel directly along this path, increasing the chances of getting hit cleanly. The key is to constantly reposition your head and body so you're not where your opponent expects you to be.

Head Movement and the Centerline

One of the most effective ways to defend yourself in the danger zone is through head movement. Slipping, bobbing and weaving take your head off the centerline, making you a more elusive target. Head movement isn't merely for defense, though, it's equally important when you're throwing punches. By slipping off the centerline, you also create openings to counter your opponent's straight punches. A well-timed slip can position you for a counter cross, hook, or body shot, allowing you to make them pay for their aggression.

If you're operating outside the danger zone, your head can remain more centered or slightly back because you're further from your opponent's range. Since straight punches travel along the centerline, the simplest way to avoid them is by staying at a distance where that centerline no longer intersects with your head's position. However, once you enter the danger zone, keeping your head on the centerline increases the risk of getting hit, making head movement essential.

By keeping your head off the centerline, you force your opponent to adjust their aim, making it harder for them to land clean shots. This split-second of adjustment gives you time to react, counter, or escape before their punch lands.

Throwing Punches While Off the Centerline

Moving your head "off line" while throwing punches is essential to avoid getting hit simultaneously, especially with committed strikes like the cross or overhand. Staying on the centerline while delivering these powerful punches leaves you open to a well-timed counter, making it crucial to shift your head off the line mid-attack.

This same principle applies when throwing the jab. Although the jab generally carries less risk than a heavier punch, slipping your head off the centerline while jabbing gives you a distinct advantage when you and your opponent are trading jabs, particularly against an opponent in the same stance (orthodox vs. orthodox or southpaw vs. southpaw). Moving your head off the line makes it harder for your opponent to land their jab cleanly, while you remain in position to land yours.

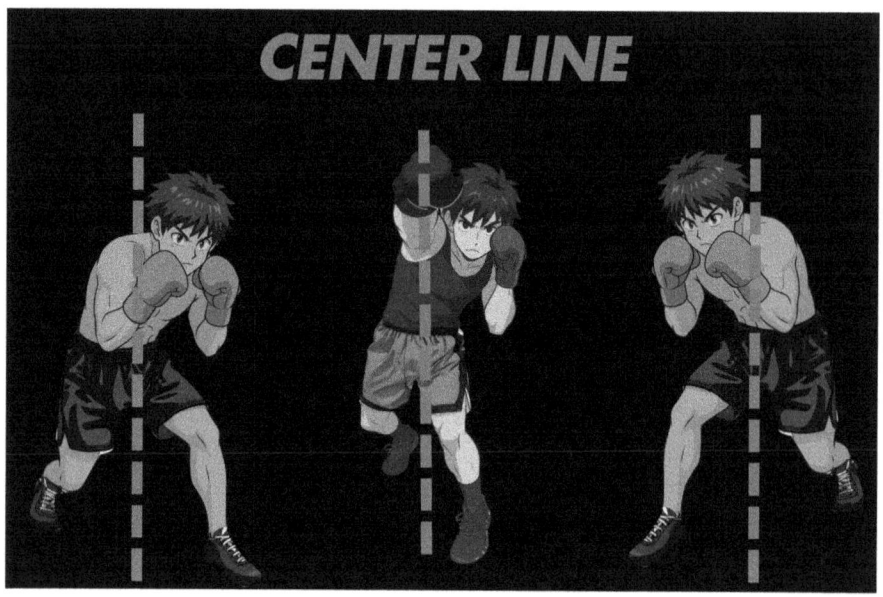

Whether you slip or step at an angle, head movement ensures you're protecting yourself while staying elusive and aggressive.

Tip: Always keep your chin down and head tucked when throwing punches off-line. This keeps you in a better defensive position as you attack.

Drills for Centerline Awareness

Slip and Strike: Practice slipping your head off the centerline as you throw punches. For example, slightly slip to the outside while throwing a jab or cross, ensuring you stay safe from counters.

Offensive Head Movement: Combine head movement with punching combinations, making sure your head shifts off the centerline. The natural rotation of your punches will move your head slightly off-line, making you safer during exchanges. At higher levels, some fighters learn to deliberately exaggerate this by slipping or rolling as they punch, blending offense and defense seamlessly. Incorporate counterpunching by slipping an imaginary jab or cross before responding with a punch of your own.

Maintaining awareness of the centerline goes beyond avoiding punches. It's about throwing with confidence, knowing you're minimizing the risk of getting hit while delivering your own shots.

The Snap: Whipping Your Punches for Maximum Impact

One of the most effective techniques is learning how to whip your punches. Imagine your fist as a ball and your arm as the string, when thrown correctly, the energy flows smoothly from your base through your arm, generating speed before snapping forward with impact. Think of a small ball attached to a loose rope being snapped forward, the way a fisherman flicks a cast. The key is allowing your arm to stay loose and fluid until the last instant, when the energy whips through and explodes on impact.

This section explains how to whip your punches for maximum power and effectiveness.

The Mechanics of Whipping Your Punches

Relaxation is Key

Staying relaxed is necessary for a proper energy transfer. The more relaxed you are, the faster and stronger your punches will be. Power comes from the "snap" of the punch, where all the energy is transferred on impact.

Whip Like a Towel

Think of whipping a towel, the force and speed come from a flick, not from tensing your muscles. Keep your hands slightly open and clench into a tight fist right at the moment of impact. Power comes from a combination of speed and strength (in physics terms, mass × acceleration). This technique ensures all the energy is transferred at the "snap" of the punch.

Extend Your Arm

Fully extend your arm to focus the energy at the point of impact. The momentum builds up, and the power is delivered right at the snap. For straight punches, full extension ensures maximum reach and power transfer. However, hooks and uppercuts generate their snap differently, relying more on the arc and the sharp rotation of the body.

Relaxed Shoulders

Keep your shoulders relaxed to prevent losing power. As you improve, you'll naturally develop a subtle 'shoulder snap' that adds extra sharpness to all of your punches, including hooks and uppercuts, without telegraphing your moves. Staying loose in your shoulders helps you maintain fluidity and speed.

The Gas and Brake Principle

If you tense up during your punch, it's like pressing both the gas and brake pedals at the same time, your speed and power will be limited. Instead, stay relaxed and only tense your muscles at the moment of impact. This assures all the energy is transferred to your opponent, making your punches much more effective.

The Kinetic Chain: From Legs to Torso

The power in your punch comes from the ground up, known as the kinetic chain:

- **Legs:** The punch begins with a strong push off the ground.
- **Torso:** Power flows through the quick rotation of your torso.
- **Arms**: Finally, the energy transfers to your arms and releases at the snap of your punch.

Effortless Potency

Whipping your punches increases their power without using extra energy. This technique allows you to maintain your stamina while still delivering strong punches. By staying relaxed, you make your punches faster, and stronger, without tiring yourself out.

Tips for Perfecting the Snap

Practice Relaxation: Stay loose and relaxed until the moment of impact. Shadowbox with a focus on relaxation.

Work on Timing: Perfect your timing by clenching your fist at the exact moment of impact. Practice on a heavy bag or pads to fine-tune this.

Use Visualizations: Visualize your punches as a ball at the end of a string to help understand the fluid motion required.

Stretch Regularly: Keep your muscles flexible and loose through regular stretching and mobility exercises.

Focus on Technique: Work with a coach to continuously progress your form and technique.

Chapter 4
Footwork Finesse

"Float like a butterfly, sting like a bee." [7]
—Muhammad Ali

As Ali so famously said, effective footwork allows you to control the fight with grace. Footwork is the foundation of success in boxing. It's about understanding space, staying balanced, and dictating the pace of the fight. Skilled footwork allows you to create openings, avoid your opponent's strikes, and maintain control in the ring. These techniques can be practiced in the ring or in any suitable space to develop real-time skills that translate directly to fight scenarios.

Few fighters embodied the art of footwork like Willie Pep. Known for his elusive movement, Pep once famously won a round without throwing a single punch, relying solely on his masterful footwork and defensive skills to neutralize his opponent. His ability to control a fight with his legs alone highlights the importance of developing exceptional footwork as a cornerstone of your boxing style.

Key Footwork Techniques (and Drills)

Forward and Backward Movement

Controlling distance is crucial in a fight, and proper footwork allows you to stay balanced while adjusting your position. Moving forward helps you close the gap and apply pressure, while stepping backward allows you to create space and evade attacks without compromising your stance. Having superior distance control will give you a significant advantage over your opponent. Fighters who can manage range effectively can dictate

---

[7] Ali, Muhammad. Quote from pre-fight interview before the Rumble in the Jungle bout against George Foreman, Kinshasa, Zaïre (now Democratic Republic of the Congo), October 30, 1974.

when exchanges happen, force opponents into uncomfortable positions, and make them hesitant to commit.

Drill It: Practice stepping forward and backward while keeping your stance intact. When moving forward, take a short step with your lead foot, and your rear foot follows by moving the same distance, if your lead foot moves four inches, your back foot moves four inches. The same applies when stepping backward; your rear foot moves first, and your lead foot follows, covering the exact distance to maintain balance. Keep your movements controlled and precise, avoiding unnecessary weight shifts or overextending. This drill can be practiced through shadowboxing or with a partner to reinforce proper footwork in realistic scenarios.

Cutting Off the Ring

Mastering this technique allows you to control your opponent's movement, forcing them into corners or against the ropes, where their options are limited. By cutting off escape routes, you create opportunities to apply pressure, set traps, and capitalize on their mistakes.

Drill It: Whether shadowboxing or working with a partner, practice cutting off your opponent's movement by stepping laterally to the left or right, mirroring their motion to close off their exits. Instead of chasing, angle your footwork to block their path and force them into a confined space where you can dictate the action. Stay alert, balanced, and ready to strike when they have nowhere left to go.

In-and-Out Footwork & Pendulum Step

Think of this as a rhythm: you glide in and out of range smoothly, controlling the distance between you and your opponent. This technique strengthens your legs and conditions your body until you can do this effortlessly. Think of fighters like Manny Pacquiao and Dmitry Bivol, who use in-and-out footwork to throw off their opponents' timing. They surge in for quick strikes and slip back out before their opponents even know what hit them. The pendulum step is a useful variation of in-and-out footwork, where you shift your weight forward by stepping lightly with your lead foot while your back foot follows naturally, then rock back by reversing the motion, maintaining a smooth, controlled rhythm.

Drill It: Practice moving in and out, focusing on stepping forward to close the gap and back out to avoid counters. Incorporate the pendulum step to add fluidity to your motion, allowing you to control range while staying balanced and ready to counter. This drill builds endurance and conditioning necessary to do it effectively in a fight.

Lateral Movement

Lateral movement keeps you elusive by allowing you to move side to side, forcing your opponent to constantly adjust. It's key for staying unpredictable while creating openings for attack. The mechanics are similar to forward and backward movement: each step is matched by the other foot to maintain balance and positioning. When stepping to the left, your right foot follows. When stepping to the right, your left foot follows.

Common Mistake: Crossing Your Feet

Crossing your feet while moving laterally can throw off your balance and leave you open to counters. It's a risky habit, especially for beginners. Focus on controlled shuffles to maintain stability.

Drill It: Practice lateral movement, focusing on quick, controlled shuffles left and right while maintaining balance and stance.

Pivoting

Pivoting allows you to quickly create new angles for attack or defense by rotating on your lead foot. It's essential for adjusting your position while maintaining balance.

Drill It: Imagine your lead foot is drilled into the ground by a nail, anchoring you in place. As you pivot, your back foot swivels naturally around **it**, allowing you to rotate left or right while maintaining your stance. Your back foot may slide or slightly lift to adjust, but your lead foot remains your pivot point. Pivots help open up fresh angles for counters.

Shifting (Advanced Technique)

Shifting is an advanced stance-switching technique where you punch while moving your back foot forward, transitioning into a new stance. It confuses opponents and helps close the distance quickly. Fighters like Jack Dempsey, Dmitry Pirog and Marvin Hagler used this method at times while applying pressure. Once you've shifted, you're in a new stance, ready to continue attacking without breaking momentum.

Drill It: Practice shifting by stepping your back foot forward as you throw a punch, fluidly switching stances. This can be done in the ring or any training area. Follow up with combinations to catch your opponent off-guard and seamlessly continue your offense from the new stance.

D'Amato Shift

The D'Amato Shift, named after the renowned trainer Cus D'Amato, is a dynamic footwork technique designed to create advantageous angles for offense and defense. It's a hallmark of the peek-a-boo boxing style, famously utilized by fighters like Mike Tyson.

How to do it:

1. **Initiate the Shift:** Slip to the left or right, shifting your weight onto your lead leg. This movement loads your body for the shift and helps you evade an incoming punch.

2. **Execute the Footwork:** With a smooth hop-like slide, shift your weight and reposition your feet. Your rear foot glides into a new position while your lead foot kicks out to adjust your stance. The motion should be fluid, not a full jump — your feet stay close to the ground while shifting into the new angle.

3. **Reposition for Attack:** The shift moves you off your opponent's centerline, opening up fresh angles for offense while making it difficult for them to counter.

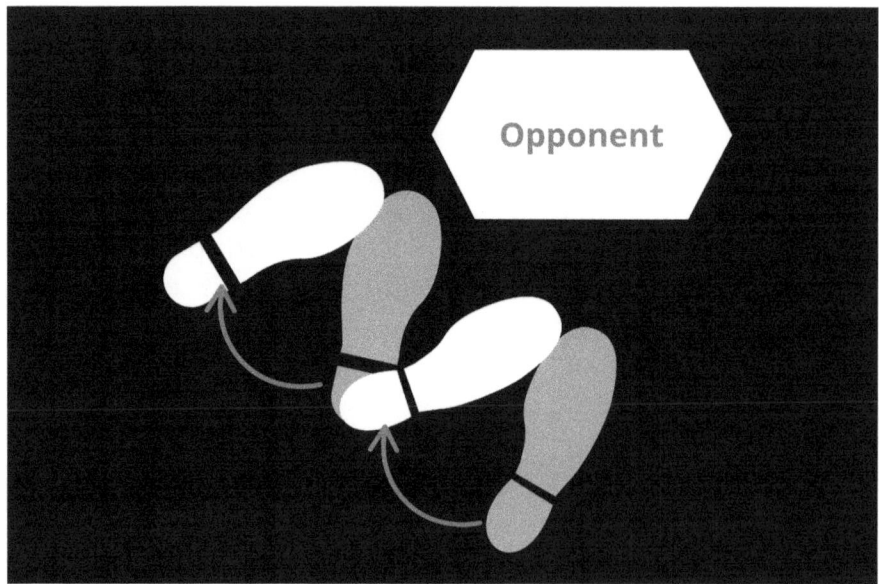

Agility Drills as Tools to Enhance Footwork

Agility drills like ladder and cone drills are useful tools for developing coordination, speed and rhythm that complement real fight scenarios.

Ladder Drills

Fighters like Nonito Donaire and Manny Pacquiao have used ladder drills to develop rapid foot movement and coordination.

High Knees Drill: Run through the ladder while lifting your knees high to develop leg strength and explosiveness.

In-and-Out Drill: Step in and out of the ladder rungs quickly, practicing controlled footwork to manage distance.

Lateral Shuffle Drill: Move sideways through the ladder to sharpen lateral footwork, essential for dodging punches and setting up counters.

Single-Leg Hop (In-and-Out): Hop in and out along the ladder on one leg, alternating between rungs. This drill improves balance and strength, especially in your lead or rear leg, conditioning you for quick footwork and stability during direction changes.

Cone Drills

Cone drills teach quick directional changes, helping fighters react swiftly in fight-like conditions.

Zig-Zag Drill: Set up cones in a zig-zag pattern and move through them, focusing on sharp direction changes. This drill helps you adjust angles, close gaps, and evade pressure.

T-Drill: Arrange cones in a T-shape. Sprint forward, side shuffle to each side, and backpedal. This helps develop multi-directional speed, essential for lateral movement and positioning.

Transferring Footwork Skills to Real Fight Scenarios

Performing drills alone isn't enough; the key is integrating these footwork exercises into your fight training. While many drills can be practiced outside the ring, their purpose is to ensure that your footwork is fluid, responsive and effective in actual fights. Every drill you practice should directly enhance your ability to move in real-time, whether shadowboxing, sparring, or during a match.

Shadowboxing

Shadowboxing is the best way to practice your footwork without the pressure of an opponent. It allows you to focus on your movement—working on balance, control and smooth transitions.

Visualize the Fight: Picture an opponent in front of you. Move in and out of range, using lateral steps and pivots to create angles and keep control of the distance.

Practice Techniques: Focus on footwork for entire rounds, performing In-and-Out steps and lateral movement. This builds the habit of using these techniques in fight situations, making them second nature.

Sparring

This is where you put your footwork to the test against a live opponent. It's where you can see how well you can time your movements, control distance, and adjust your positioning.

Fight Simulation: Move continuously, using lateral footwork, pivots and In-and-Out steps to stay unpredictable and maintain control. Focus on how your footwork can help you set up punches, create angles and avoid incoming shots.

Heavy Bag Work

When working on the heavy bag, footwork should accompany your punches. Instead of standing still, practice moving around the bag as if it's an opponent, using footwork to find better angles and position.

Proven by the Greats

Footwork drills have been a fundamental part of the training for boxing legends. Fighters like Roy Jones Jr. did numerous drills, developing footwork that made him elusive and dominant. Andre Ward has been known to say "the feet are the first line of defense", emphasizing that old-school teachers often taught "feet first". These methods have been tested and refined over decades, there's no need to overcomplicate it. By developing these movements, your footwork will naturally evolve, becoming much more effective in the ring.

Chapter 5
The Shield of Defense

"Hit and Don't Get Hit." [8]

Defense is just as important as offense. The ability to avoid getting hit while setting up your own attacks defines a complete fighter. A big part of defense is understanding that punches are always coming back, offense and defense are intertwined. Great fighters use techniques like head movement, footwork, blocking, rolling, counterpunching and clinching to avoid punishment and create opportunities. In this chapter, we'll explore the five main lines of defense, how they work, when to use them, and the techniques needed to keep yourself safe while staying ready to counterattack.

The Five Lines of Defense

Defense in boxing follows five key lines (footwork, parries, head movements, blocking and shoulder rolls, and clinching), each giving you a way to manage incoming attacks. The earlier lines focus on avoiding punches entirely, while the later ones allow you to control the impact when contact is unavoidable. No fight is the same, so you'll need to adapt, switching between these defenses depending on the situation in the ring.

Footwork—Staying Out of Range: The first and safest line of defense is footwork. By stepping out of range or pivoting to the side, you make your opponent miss completely. This forces them to reset, allowing you to control the fight's pace and create openings for counters on your own terms.

Parries—Redirecting the Attack: When movement alone isn't enough, parrying comes into play. A quick, well-timed parry deflects the punch just enough to throw off your opponent's rhythm, giving you a moment to strike back. Parries

---

[8] Traditional boxing maxim, commonly attributed to early lightweight champion Joe Gans and echoed by trainers throughout boxing history. This phrase embodies one of the sport's most fundamental principles.

require precision but keep you in range, offering a great opportunity to counter while staying protected.

Head Movement—Slipping, Bobbing/Weaving: In close-range exchanges, head movement becomes your go-to defense. Techniques like slipping (moving your head slightly off the punch's line), and bobbing and weaving (a fluid "U" motion with your upper body) allow you to avoid clean shots. Another effective method is the *Pull Back*, where you quickly pull your head just out of range to make an opponent's punch fall short. This is especially useful against straight punches but requires precise timing to avoid leaning too far and exposing yourself to follow-ups.

Blocking & Shoulder-roll—Absorbing and Countering: Blocking offers reliable protection by using your gloves, arms and shoulders to absorb punches. It allows you to stay composed under pressure and can be highly effective for setting up counters. Fighters who excel at blocking don't just absorb punches. They use the moment as a foundation to bait opponents into overcommitting, creating opportunities to return fire. While blocked punches still carry some impact, this defense helps you stay in range, ready to respond with crisp counters.

A well-timed block can also help you "roll with the punch"—using your glove, arm, or shoulder to move in the same direction as the strike. This subtle movement reduces the punch's force, softens the blow, and positions you for an immediate counter. When blocking, cuff the ear and turn in the direction the punch is coming, loading up for the return.

Extra—Advanced Head Turn (Glide Defense): Another way to minimize damage is the quick head turn—angling your chin just enough to let a punch glide past instead of absorbing full impact. This subtle move, seen in fighters like Canelo Alvarez, acts as a subtle defensive reflex in those final milliseconds before impact. It requires precision and repetition, so it should be drilled slowly before increasing speed. With enough practice, it can become second nature.

The Last Line of Defense—Clinching: When all other defensive options fail or when you need to negate your opponent's offense, clinching becomes the last line of defense. A well-executed clinch can prevent an opponent from attacking up close, allowing you to control the pace and reset the fight on your terms. Clinching is also a valuable survival tool. If you're hurt or rocked by a punch, it can buy you the time needed to recover and survive until the next bell. Fighters often use clinching strategically to disrupt aggressive opponents, forcing them to work harder while conserving their own energy. Beyond defense, clinching can also serve as an offensive tool, wearing down opponents by making them carry weight, draining their stamina as the fight progresses.

Switching between these defenses is key to staying elusive and effective. Some moments require swift footwork to avoid danger, while other situations call for tight blocking to withstand and counter. By combining these lines of defense, you make it harder for your opponent to anticipate your movements and stay in control of the fight.

Tip: When retreating, don't take more than two steps back without changing the angle. Taking more than two steps going straight back will generally put you on the ropes or into a corner where you are at a compromised position.

Anticipatory Defense

Great defense is not limited to reacting. It's about anticipating what's coming next and integrating it into your offense. If you know your opponent tends to counter with a specific punch after you throw a certain shot, you can preemptively defend against it without waiting to see if it happens.

For example, if your opponent always fires a counter hook when you throw a right cross, don't wait to see if they throw it—roll under immediately after your shot. If they throw the hook, you've already avoided it. If they don't, you're still in a safe position, ready to reset or follow up with your own attack.

Over time, you'll also develop a feel for what punches are likely to come next in a sequence. For instance, after a jab-cross, a hook—or another lead-hand variant—is often the natural follow-up. Recognizing these patterns allows you to anticipate rather than just react, making it seem like you have unreal reflexes. This instinct doesn't come from luck. It comes from repetition, constantly seeing and feeling punches in training until recognizing these sequences becomes second nature.

Train yourself to be ready for multiple sequences, not only one. Fighters often get caught on the second or third exchange, not because they lack skill, but because they haven't conditioned themselves to instinctively handle combinations beyond the first. Always finish every sequence on defense, staying alert for any trailing shots until the full exchange has played out.

Anticipatory defense also allows you to stay one step ahead. Whether it's automatically slipping after a jab, rolling after a right hand, or pivoting after a combination, this type of proactive defense keeps you safe while allowing you to capitalize on mistakes the moment they happen.

Defensive Styles and Techniques

Each line of defense can be applied through different styles, giving fighters multiple ways to protect themselves and counterattack. Some fighters prefer specific styles, while others blend them to keep their opponents guessing.

Philly Shell/Shoulder Roll

Fits under: Head Movement and Blocking

How to do it: Tuck your chin behind your lead shoulder, using your rear hand to block or catch punches. Your lead arm rests low, shielding your body while staying ready to parry or counter. This style frustrates opponents by making clean shots difficult to land. Angle your lead shoulder to deflect punches off it, redirecting their force and minimizing damage. Fighters like James Toney and Floyd Mayweather Jr. used the Philly Shell to deflect punches while staying ready to counter.

High Guard

Fits under: Blocking

How to do it: Raising both hands to cover your head and face offers solid protection against straight punches. Fighters like Winky Wright and Errol Spence Jr. have used the high guard while applying pressure on opponents, blending defense with aggressive offense.

Long Guard

Fits under: Parries and Blocking

How to do it: Extending your lead hand outward helps control the distance, while the rear hand stays close to your chin for protection. This guard is effective for parrying and intercepting straight punches, and the extended arm can also act as a shield to block hooks. Larry Holmes used this style to keep opponents at bay with his jab, but overextending the lead hand can leave you open to counters. I recommend stepping back at the same time as blocking punches with the long guard, if you stay stationary, punches can loop around your extended arm and target the body or head.

Cross Guard

Fits under: Blocking

How to do it: In this style, the rear hand crosses over the face, shielding the opposite side of the head, while the lead hand rests lower across the body, covering the ribs. This creates a strong defensive shell against both head and body shots. Archie Moore was known for using the cross guard to absorb punches and create openings for counters, though it can limit vision. This defense has become more uncommon in modern boxing, but it remains a valuable tool in the right hands, especially when mastered through repetition and paired with sharp counterattacks.

Reverse Cross Guard

Fits under: Blocking

How to do it: This variation positions the lead arm across the face, covering the opposite side, while the rear arm stays lower, closer to the chest or ribs, allowing for quicker offensive transitions. Ken Norton effectively used the reverse cross guard to disrupt opponents, though sharp timing is necessary due to limited visibility. Like the cross guard, this defense is also less common today.

Tips for Staying Safe

- **Defense Creates Counter Opportunities:** Good defense is more than avoiding punches , it's about positioning yourself to take advantage of your opponent's mistakes. Every slip, block, or parry is an opportunity to counter.

- **Why Keep Your Chin Down:** Tucking your chin minimizes the target area and protects your jaw from knockout punches. An exposed chin makes you more vulnerable to clean hits, increasing the risk of getting knocked out.

- **Keep Your Eyes on the Chest and Opponent:** One useful tip is to focus on the opponent's chest. It can help you see punches coming without lifting your chin, keeping you safer from unexpected shots. At the same time, this will give you awareness of their movements to read attacks and set up your own counters.

Common Mistakes

Relying too heavily on one line of defense or becoming predictable makes it easier for your opponent to read your movements. The best fighters mix their defenses, switching between footwork, parrying, head movement, blocking and clinching to keep their opponents off balance. Ignoring clinching as a defensive tool can leave you vulnerable up close, especially against pressure fighters. By staying dynamic, you become harder to hit and more dangerous with each counter.

How to Escape the Clinch

While clinching can be an effective way to control a fight, knowing how to escape the clinch is just as important. If an opponent locks you up, you need to break free quickly to regain control. Here are some key ways to escape:

1. **Frame and Push Off:** Place your forearm or hand against your opponent's shoulder, collarbone, or face, then press and step back to create space.

2. **Use Footwork to Pivot Out:** Instead of fighting force with force, turn your body at an angle to slip out of the clinch while staying in a position to counter.

3. **Hand-Fighting and Breaking Grips:** Peel your opponent's arms away by digging inside their grip, controlling their wrist or elbow, and using quick lateral movement to break free.

4. **Hit While One Arm is Trapped:** If your opponent manages to hold one of your arms, use your free hand to strike with short uppercuts, hooks, or body shots to force them to loosen their grip.

Defensive Drill

Practice the five lines of defense with a partner using light punches. Take turns stepping out of range, parrying, slipping, blocking, and clinching when necessary to control distance and shut down inside attacks. This drill helps you transition smoothly between defenses, building muscle memory for live fights. Repeating these movements at different levels of intensity will prepare you to handle the variety of challenges you'll face in the ring. We'll cover more advanced drills in a later chapter.

Chapter 6
How Boxing Matches Are Scored:
A Complete Guide

"Perception is reality." [9]
—Lee Atwater, famed political strategist

Landing punches alone won't win the fight; it's about convincing the judges that you're in control. Whether in professional or amateur bouts, understanding the scoring system and how to influence judges gives you a competitive edge. Beyond technical skill, body language and demeanor can sway close rounds in your favor. In this chapter, we'll cover the rules, key criteria judges use, and how both physical and psychological strategies can help you win on the scorecards.

The 10-Point Must System

Professional boxing uses the 10-point must system to score each round. The winning fighter gets 10 points, and the opponent typically receives 9. Here's how scores are adjusted:

Winning the Round: The fighter who guides the flow of the fight and lands cleaner punches wins 10-9.

Knockdowns: Each knockdown drops the other fighter's score by a point (e.g., 10-8). Multiple knockdowns may result in a 10-7 score.

Draw Rounds: If neither fighter gains an edge, judges may score the round 10-10.

Fouls: Referees can deduct points for infractions like low blows or hitting after the bell.

---

[9] Atwater, Lee. Political strategist and Republican campaign advisor. Quote reflecting his philosophy on political messaging and public perception, widely cited in political strategy contexts.

Strategic Use of Scoring Criteria

A fighter who demonstrates a balance of effective aggression, ring generalship, clean punches, and defense leaves a strong impression on judges. By consciously addressing each of these criteria during the fight, you can maximize your chances of winning close rounds.

1. Effective Aggression

Moving forward or looking to force the action with intelligent offense while avoiding getting hit.

Why it matters: Judges favor fighters who appear to be in charge of the action. Taking the lead and making your opponent react shows control.

How to apply:

- Be active, but don't attack recklessly. Land meaningful punches while staying defensively responsible.
- Use consistent pressure to push your opponent back and dictate where the fight takes place.
- Even when you're not landing clean punches, forcing your opponent to react to your movement or feints demonstrates you are controlling the fight.

2. Ring Generalship

The ability to control the pace, positioning and flow of the fight —forcing your opponent to react to you.

Why it matters: Controlling the fight's pace and positioning shows dominance. Judges notice when one fighter dictates the terms of the fight.

How to apply:

- Control the center of the ring and force your opponent to move on your terms.
- Make the fight happen where you're strongest, whether that's inside, at mid-range, or long range.

- Avoid predictability. Change your rhythm and angles to keep your opponent guessing and reactive.

3. Clean Punches Landed

Only solid hits to the head, face, or upper body count. Glancing blows don't.

Why it matters: Clean, effective punches that land with impact carry significant weight with many judges. Judges notice punches that are sharp and intentional, and these often make the biggest impression when scoring close rounds.

How to apply:

- Prioritize punches that land solidly and clearly over glancing blows. It's not just about how many punches you throw, it's about making them count.

- Use combinations strategically. Even if not every shot lands clean, one or two well-placed punches in the sequence can catch the judge's eye.

- Aim for visible targets like the head or ribs, as punches that land in noticeable areas are more likely to influence scoring.

4. Defense

Slipping, blocking, or evading punches demonstrates high-level skill.

Why it matters: Judges respect fighters who avoid damage while staying active. Defense showcases skill and composure.

How to apply:

- Make your opponent miss in a way that's obvious to the judges. Big misses highlight your defensive ability.

- Use your defense to set up counters. A well-timed counter after slipping or blocking a punch shows control.

- Stay composed while defending. A calm, controlled fighter projects confidence, even under pressure.

Appeal to All Judges: The Balanced Approach

By showing a mix of aggression, ring control, clean punches and defense throughout the fight, you appeal to judges regardless of their individual biases. Even if one judge leans toward aggression and another favors defense or clean punching, you'll have elements that resonate with all.

Body Language: Creating the Perception of Control in the Ring

Winning on the scorecards is more than physical dominance; you have to *look* like the winner. Judges, whether they realize it or not, respond to body language. That's where the Reticular Activating System (RAS) comes in—the brain's built-in filter for what stands out or matches expectations. It might sound a little science-y, but here's what matters: when you look composed, confident and in control, you naturally draw more attention. In close rounds, that perception alone can tip the scoring in your favor.

Practical Body Language Strategies for Control

Below are key strategies used by elite fighters to maintain the perception of control. These tactics not only sway the judges but also subtly affect your opponent, causing hesitation and doubt.

1. Stay Relaxed Under Pressure

Why it Matters: Tension signals discomfort and makes you look overwhelmed. A relaxed fighter projects calmness and control.

How to Apply: Keep your shoulders loose, avoid clenching your fists between punches, and let your movements stay fluid. This conserves energy and also makes you harder to read.

2. Control Facial Expressions

Why it Matters: Facial expressions send powerful signals. Fighters like Miguel Cotto are known for maintaining stoic expressions throughout a fight, revealing little to no emotion. This makes it nearly impossible for opponents—or judges, to gauge their fatigue or pain. Others, like Floyd Mayweather, use subtle gestures, such as shaking their head or even saying 'nope,' to dismiss their opponent's punches and suggest they had no effect.

How to Apply: Stay calm after taking a clean shot. Whether you prefer a neutral, unreadable expression or calculated nonverbal cues to downplay your opponent's attacks, these actions create doubt about your opponent's effectiveness and assure judges that you're in control.

3. Quick Recovery After Taking a Hit

Why it Matters: Reacting poorly to a punch makes the hit appear more damaging. Recovering quickly after being hit signals toughness and resilience, reassuring judges that you are unfazed.

How to Apply: When hit, immediately reset your stance, maintain posture, and make eye contact with your opponent. This will send the message that you're still in control.

4. Maintain Frame Between Rounds

Why it Works: Your demeanor during breaks reveals your stamina and mental state. Fighters who look calm between rounds project endurance and confidence.

How to Apply: Walk to your corner calmly. Sit upright, control your breathing, and maintain eye contact with your team. Avoid slumping or gasping for air, even if you feel tired. This helps you appear steady and assured throughout the fight.

5. Feign Indifference to Your Opponent's Success

Why it Matters: Showing frustration or anger after your opponent lands punches can shift the psychological edge in their favor.

How to Apply: Keep your responses minimal after taking a clean shot, whether it's a quick shake of the head, or simply remaining neutral. These cues can frustrate your opponent and reassure judges that the punch was insignificant.

6. Project Control by Initiating Exchanges

Why it Matters: Judges favor fighters who dictate the fight's pace. Even if an exchange is even, the fighter who initiates it often looks like the aggressor.

How to Apply: Start each exchange with a purposeful jab or feint to set the rhythm. Make your opponent react to you, not the other way around.

7. Maintain Focus After a Clean Shot

Why it Works: Judges are more likely to favor fighters who stay composed and focused after landing a punch. Overreacting to a successful hit can suggest immaturity or loss of control, while calm behavior reinforces the impression that you expect to be winning.

How to Apply: After landing a clean punch, keep your posture steady, don't celebrate or overreact. Stay locked in, and be ready to continue controlling the fight.

The A-Side and B-Side

How Confirmation Bias can Affect Judging and Opponents

In professional boxing, fighters are often divided into an A-side and a B-side. The A-side is usually the bigger name or the favorite, coming into the fight with higher expectations. Judges, like anyone else, are prone to confirmation bias—the tendency to interpret new information in ways that support what they already believe or expect.

If the judges expect the A-side to win, they may unconsciously give more weight to their actions, even if the B-side performs just as well. However, a B-side fighter who projects confidence, stays composed, and controls key moments can shift the judges' focus and disrupt expectations. This demeanor also influences the opponent, causing hesitation and discomfort, which opens opportunities for the B-side fighter to take over.

Final Thought: Control Both the Fight and Its Perception

Winning a boxing match isn't solely about physical skill; it's a balance of strategy, execution, and presentation. When the fight is close, judges look beyond who lands more punches. They assess who appears to be in control, who dictates the action, and who looks like the winner.

Use the scoring system to your advantage by showcasing a mix of effective aggression, ring generalship, clean punches, and defense in every round. Pair this with confident body language and a commanding presence that leaves no room for doubt. Whether you're the A-side or B-side, remember that controlling both the fight and its perception can tip the scorecards in your favor.

Round 2: Advanced Fight Craft

Chapter 7
Boxing IQ: There Are Levels to This

"Strategy without tactics is the slowest route to victory.
Tactics without strategy is the noise before defeat." [10]
—Sun Tzu, author of The Art of War

Boxing IQ goes far beyond knowing how to throw or dodge punches. It's about reading your opponent, anticipating their moves, and reacting effectively. Imagine facing an opponent who is taller, faster, or stronger. A high boxing IQ allows you to turn their strengths into weaknesses. By using feints or superior footwork, you can control the fight's pace and take advantage of openings.

Developing a high boxing IQ takes time, but with dedication and practice, you can increase your ability to read and react in the ring. This advanced understanding of the sport allows some boxers to transcend weight classes and win titles in multiple divisions. Their ability to adapt, strategize and outthink opponents at different weights highlights the true power of a high boxing IQ.

Boxing IQ means understanding what to do, when to do it, and why. In the next chapters, we'll break down the skills that take fight intelligence to the next level: the art of counterpunching, mastering deception through feints, controlling rhythm, and setting traps that force your opponent into mistakes.

The Craft of the Counterpunch

"Make 'em miss, make 'em pay." [11]

Counterpunching is a key weapon that lets you capitalize on your opponent's missed punches and exploit their moments of vulnerability. A well-placed counter can instantly shift the

---

[10] Sun Tzu, "The Art of War," Chapter 5: Energy, circa 5th century BCE. Translated by Lionel Giles (1910).

[11] Traditional boxing axiom. A fundamental principle of counter-punching taught in boxing gyms worldwide.

momentum in your favor, and there are several options at your disposal.

Catch Counter: This involves blocking your opponent's punch and immediately firing back, either with the same arm you used to block or the opposite one. For instance, if your opponent throws a hook, you block it with your glove (known as 'catching'), then quickly counter with an uppercut to the body or a hook to the head. This technique interrupts their attack and sets up a strong counterpunch opportunity. A classic example is catching a jab with your rear hand and immediately firing back with your own jab, helping you stay in control of the battle of the jabs.

Parry Counter: This counter uses redirection rather than absorption. Instead of blocking or slipping the punch, you quickly deflect it, usually with your lead or rear hand, to send it off course and immediately fire back. For example, if your opponent throws a jab, you can parry it inward with your rear hand and follow up with a straight right or sharp lead hook.

Slip Counter: You slip your opponent's punch by moving your head off the centerline and immediately return fire. For instance, slipping a jab and countering with a cross is a common method, or slipping to the outside of a cross and countering with a hook.

Step Back Counter: When your opponent throws a punch, you step back just enough to make them miss, then quickly counter when they're vulnerable. Stepping out of range creates space and catches your opponent off guard as they overextend.

Pull Counter: A classic and deadly move, the pull counter involves slightly leaning or pulling your upper body back to evade a punch (typically a jab) then immediately snapping back with a sharp counter, usually a right cross. This technique works well against opponents who overcommit on the jab or fall in after their shots. It punishes them for reaching and gives you a clean opening with maximum leverage.

Timing Counter: Another effective counterpunch technique is timing your opponent's punch while throwing your own. For example, as your opponent throws a cross, you can move your head slightly off the centerline and throw a short, chopping overhand right at the same time. The goal is for your punch to land while theirs misses, often having devastating effects. This requires sharp timing and accuracy, using their punch against them.

Effective counterpunching requires timing and awareness of distance. Knowing when and where to strike is crucial for success. Counterpunching demands waiting for the right moment. Rushing a counter or hesitating can leave you exposed. Trust your instincts and training to react when the time is right.

Drill It: Practice with a partner, focusing on counterpunching immediately after you slip, block, or step back from their punches. Incorporate timing counters by practicing slipping or moving off line while throwing punches at the same time your partner does. Use mitt work to sharpen your timing and accuracy.

Feints: The Subtlety of Deception

"All warfare is based on deception. Hence, when we are able to attack, we must seem unable; when using our forces, we must appear inactive; when we are near, we must make the enemy believe we are far away; when far away, we must make him believe we are near."[12] — Sun Tzu, The Art of War

In boxing, as in war, not every move is meant to land. Feinting is an art of deception, a small gesture or movement that keeps your opponent guessing, giving you control over the rhythm of the fight. At its core, a feint looks like a real punch but isn't. It's a calculated bluff meant to draw a reaction, create hesitation, or set the trap for the shot that truly matters. It's a master's tool that opens doors and exposes weaknesses, letting you slip through your opponent's guard with subtlety rather than brute force.

---

[12] Sun Tzu, "The Art of War," Chapter 1: Laying Plans, Verse 18-19. Translated by Lionel Giles (1910). Originally written circa 5th century BCE.

Why Feints Are Necessary in Boxing

Feints are a must, especially as you reach higher levels and face more experienced opponents. At these stages, avoiding predictable movements is critical. Skilled fighters can read even well-executed punches, making it essential to use feints to keep them guessing.

When your opponent is forced to react to a mix of real attacks and feints, it opens them up for effective counters.

Using feints keeps your opponent attuned to your rhythm, which inevitably opens them up for attacks. Imagine you feint a jab, and your opponent reacts. This tells you how they might respond to a real jab, and also reveals openings you can exploit. You can then mix in more feints to keep them off-balance. And if they eventually stop reacting, that too can create its own kind of opportunity.

The Psychology of Feinting

The beauty of a feint is that it gets inside the opponent's head. When you make them react to something that isn't real, you're already one step ahead. By forcing them to play your game, you wear them down mentally, steal their focus, and plant seeds of hesitation. Feints keep your opponent's mind occupied, putting them in a constant state of reaction while you dictate the pace of the fight. When they're focused on responding to your every move, it becomes difficult for them to mentally organize their own offense. Even the smallest movements, a quick twitch, a light shift, or a slight step, can give them the impression you're coming in hard when you're actually just testing their reactions.

What Makes a Good Feint?

A good feint is more than just a casual flick or weak gesture; it has to look convincing and deliberate. High-level boxers know that lazy or uncommitted feints won't fool skilled opponents. The best feints mirror the exact mechanics of a real punch or movement, making it challenging for the opponent to spot the difference. Fighters like Floyd Mayweather mastered this by using small, sharp movements that are so believable, opponents feel compelled to react, because they know his real punches are fast, precise, and hard to evade.

The difference between a good and a poor feint often comes down to speed, timing and believability. A telegraphed or slow feint won't provoke a reaction from an experienced opponent. To make your feints effective, focus on building speed, accuracy, and the ability to make even slight movements feel threatening. Feints don't have to be large to be convincing, they just have to feel real enough to keep your opponent guessing.

Types of Feints

Feints come in many forms. Some are subtle, some are bold, and each serves a different strategic purpose. Whether it's with your hands, feet, head, or overall rhythm, the goal is the same: to draw a reaction, create an opening, or disrupt your opponent's timing. Understanding the different types of feints expands your ability to manipulate the fight on your terms.

Hand Feints

Hand feints are about throwing "almost punches" that trigger defensive reactions without full commitment. One classic example is the *jab feint*, where you snap a quick jab but pull it back at the last moment, often causing your opponent to flinch and expose their defensive habits.

One hand feint I sharpened while working with legendary trainer Jesse Reid, who coached 29 world champions, involves keeping both hands in motion in front of the opponent. By using these hand feints, you create a steady engagement that's hard to ignore. Fighters like Oleksandr Usyk use a similar approach, constantly moving their lead hand to keep the opponent unsettled. This forces the opponent to stay engaged, creating a constant threat that demands their attention. When combined with quick punches, other types of feints, and a high punch output, it becomes even more powerful. This fatigues the opponent with a relentless pace, deceptive signals and unpredictable timing, keeping them mentally on edge and making it harder for them to anticipate your next move.

The Throw-Away Feint

Canelo Alvarez has perfected this crafty move. The throw-away feint involves a quick flick of one hand, usually away from the target. It looks like a lazy punch to the side but serves a clever purpose, it draws the opponent's guard out of position, giving you a split-second opening to strike with the opposite hand. By drawing their focus with a meaningless gesture, you set up your real shot where they least expect it.

Footwork Feints

Footwork feints use subtle, quick movements to keep opponents off-balance and unsure of timing or distance.

Stutter-Step Feint: Fighters like Manny Pacquiao and Keith Thurman are both known for the stutter-step feint, though they use it in slightly different ways. Pacquiao's stutter-step is explosive, using rapid shuffles to create unpredictable timing and catch opponents off guard. Thurman, on the other hand, uses it to bait reactions, keeping opponents tense and unsure of his next move. By breaking their natural rhythm, the stutter step makes it hard for the opponent to anticipate the real attack.

In-and-Out Feint: Dmitry Bivol is a master of the in-and-out feint, using a quick bounce forward and back to manipulate distance. By stepping in and pulling back quickly, he creates a false sense of range, often causing opponents to bite on the fake. This movement allows him to read their timing and step in for real attacks as they relax or overcommit.

Head and Shoulder Feints

Subtle but deadly, head and shoulder feints are great for baiting specific reactions. A simple *head fake*, a small tilt forward or to the side, can make the opponent think you're slipping into range or ducking to the body. Fighters like Vasyl Lomachenko use head feints to keep opponents constantly guessing, making it hard to tell when he'll actually commit to an attack. Lomachenko's small, quick head movements create the illusion of vulnerability or an incoming punch, causing opponents to react early and leave openings for him to exploit. The *shoulder feint* works similarly: a slight roll of the shoulder makes it seem like a punch is coming. If they bite on the fake, you're in control.

Body Feints

Body feints play with high and low levels to trigger instinctive reactions. One of the most effective is the *level change feint,* where you dip your body as if going for a body shot, often lowering your knees slightly. Fighters like Saul "Canelo" Alvarez use this to make opponents brace their guard, creating leverage to drive an uppercut up the middle or come around the guard with an explosive hook. This feint capitalizes on instinct. The moment the opponent braces or drops their hands, they've exposed themselves to a powerful shot upstairs.

Layering Feints: Taking Deception to the Next Level

A single feint can be effective, but stacking multiple feints in succession creates a deeper level of deception, making it harder for opponents to read your intentions. This is the art of layering feints, where one fake sets up another before leading into the real attack. These are examples of layered feints that can be deployed. As you develop, you can experiment and get creative with sequences that work best for you.

Triple Feint Setup: You feint a jab, no reaction. You fake a right cross with a quick hand feint, and they flinch. You feint another jab, they react—now they're primed for a real right hand they won't see coming.

Feinting a Punch into a Footwork Trap: Step in with a feinted jab, pull back as they throw their counter, then step back in with a hard counter of your own.

Feinting High to Land Low: Feint a jab to the head, then throw a real jab to the head. Follow with a right cross hand feint to continue drawing their guard high, then dig a real left hook to the body as they overreact upstairs.

Double Stutter-Step Into Jab-Cross: In classic Pacquiao fashion, use a double stutter-step feint as a false forward advance, it draws a reaction and gets the opponent anticipating pressure. Then immediately snap off a fast jab-cross combination through the center before they have time to reset.

High-Low-High Setup: Feint a jab to the head, then throw a real jab to sell the threat upstairs. Immediately drop your level as if you're going to the body, triggering a defensive drop, then drive upward with an explosive uppercut up the middle, exploiting the opening as they brace low.

Adapting Feints Based on Opponent Reaction

Your follow-up attack after a successful feint depends on how your opponent reacts. For example, if you throw a hand feint and your opponent briefly drops their hand to block the fake punch, you've learned something important about their habits. Now you can use this to your advantage: pretend to feint again, but instead of faking, throw a real hook to the area they've left open. By reading and reacting to these patterns, you can make your feints even more effective, exploiting every opening your opponent creates.

Also, each opponent will have their unique tendencies. If you're fighting someone who's uncomfortable with body shots, feinting low could create a reliable opening. You might feint a jab to the head, then suddenly drop low and rip a left hook to the liver, using their high guard against them. You can feint to provoke a specific reaction, then immediately follow with a real shot that exploits it, catching them off guard while they're still reacting to the fake. The key is reading their reactions and adjusting your feints to keep them guessing.

Disguised Intentions: Making Your Opponent Take the Bait

Once you have a solid understanding of feints, you can take them further by using your body language to hide your intentions. Instead of looking ready to attack, try to appear relaxed or even slightly unguarded, like you're not a threat in that moment. This approach can lure your opponent into attacking, thinking you're open. But the moment they move in, you're ready with a lightning-quick counter, catching them off-guard because they've fallen for the bait.

Sometimes, the opponent won't attack, but instead tries to match your energy or posture, turning the moment into a mental standoff rather than a physical exchange.

An advanced example of this technique comes from Roy Jones Jr., who famously used a "rooster" feint in his fight against James Toney. Jones dropped his hands, leaned forward with his chest out, and looked almost tauntingly relaxed, inviting Toney to strike. Rather than take the bait immediately, Toney copied the posture—replicating the exact feint—as if to challenge Jones psychologically. This type of response is more common than many realize; opponents will often instinctively respond in kind to a feint, whether to mock it or test its legitimacy. But even this kind of reaction can be used against them. Jones repeated the feint, knowing his opponent would mirror him again, this time following it up with a lightning-fast hook that caught Toney off-guard. The entire sequence unfolded over a few calculated exchanges, and this moment showed how feints can evolve across multiple exchanges, building psychological tension and setting up an opponent for the perfect shot.

How to Make Feints Effective

A great feint needs more than motion alone; it needs to be convincing. Selling a feint requires committed body language, and an understanding of when and how your opponent reacts. Here are a few tips to make your feints hit their mark:

Convincing: Fully commit to each feint as if it's a real strike.

Balanced: Maintain proper weight distribution between your feet, ensuring you stay in a ready position. This allows you to react instantly, whether following up with a real attack or adjusting based on your opponent's reaction.

Varied: Mix up feints, from jabs to footwork to body shifts. Keep your opponent off-balance by varying the timing and type of feints. Remember: feints don't win fights, landing punches does. A well-timed feint sets up a shot, but if you're constantly feinting without delivering crisp, fast punches, your opponent will catch on and stop reacting. That said, a high volume of effective feints can be a weapon in itself, that is, if your opponent respects what you're bringing. By layering feints with sharp, authoritative punches, you dictate the rhythm of the fight, control the pace, and mentally drain your opponent, forcing them to stay reactive while you stay in command.

Perceived Threat: Make your punches, in general, feel like a real danger. By throwing fast, explosive punches with intent, you create the perception of genuine risk, making your opponent much more likely to react to your feints. When every movement feels like a potential threat, they're more susceptible to responding, which opens up opportunities to capitalize.

Drills to Sharpen Your Feints

The purpose of a feint goes beyond making your opponent react; it's to understand and manipulate their reactions in real time. Find a training partner and practice different feints, paying attention to how your partner responds. Adjust your timing, add different types of feints, and see how you can use them to break down their guard and manipulate their positioning.

Speed Variation: Changing Speeds

In the battle arena, predictability can be dangerous. If your opponent gets used to your punches coming at the same speed and power, they'll be more prepared for impact and ready to exploit any mistakes. This is where the art of changing speeds comes into play. By using this technique, you'll keep your opponent guessing, create openings for powerful shots, and gain the upper hand.

Think of your punches like the ticking of a clock. If the seconds always tick at the same pace, it's easy to predict when the next tick will come. But if the clock suddenly speeds up or slows down, it throws everything off balance. In the ring, if you throw punches at a steady tempo, your opponent may get comfortable, believing they've figured out your timing. Then, suddenly switch gears, unleashing a lightning-fast combination or single shot to catch them off guard. This is the power of changing speeds, also known as throwing punches "off-rhythm".

One of the easiest and most effective ways to change speeds is by using "off-rhythm" jabs. By varying the cadence of your jabs, you not only disrupt your opponent's timing but also increase your chances of landing the jab more often and with greater accuracy.

Changing speeds disrupts your opponent's rhythm and expectations. It's like a pitcher in baseball who throws slow curveballs, then suddenly switches to a fastball, leaving the batter swinging at air. In boxing, you apply this principle by varying the speed and cadence of your punches.

Key Tips for Speed Variation

Establish a Rhythm: Start by throwing punches at a consistent tempo—slow, medium, or fast. The goal is to get your opponent used to a certain speed.

Mix It Up: After establishing a rhythm, switch things up by accelerating or slowing down at unexpected moments. You can do this with a single punch or a rapid combination after a slower series of punches.

Vary Your Power: Speed variation also includes adjusting the power behind your punches. Throw lighter, faster punches to set up a more explosive strike.

Use Feints: Feints help disguise speed changes. Throw a feint at one speed, then follow up with a real punch at a different pace.

Practice Regularly: Speed variation is a skill that requires repetition to master. Integrate these changes into your shadowboxing, bag work and sparring sessions.

Perfecting Patterns and Setups

"To become unstoppable, you must first become predictable." [13]—Kobe Bryant

Mastering the rhythm of your patterns, and then breaking them, is a key strategy for creating confusion and openings in a fight. When you "trick the brain" of your opponent, you can lead them into traps and land punches they never see coming.

I had the privilege of learning about the art of setting up opponents and breaking patterns at a high level from one of the best fighters to ever lace up the gloves, Roy Jones Jr. His approach showed me the difference between instinctively applying some of these tactics and intellectually understanding them. This opened my eyes to strategies that even seasoned fighters sometimes overlook or may not be fully aware of.

Patterns involve setting up a predictable series of movements or punches, then breaking that pattern with an unexpected attack. This technique keeps your opponents guessing and creates opportunities for powerful strikes.

Don't Wait, CREATE

Instead of waiting for an opening, you create one. Here are two distinct ways to do that:

Baiting and Countering: Rather than waiting for your opponent to make a mistake, throw punches with the intent of

---

[13] Bryant, Kobe. Quote from Mamba Sports Academy training session, circa 2018-2019. Often cited in discussions of his training philosophy and "Mamba Mentality" approach to skill development.

baiting them into countering. Once they take the bait, you counter their counter. This method relies on setting the pace and anticipating their reaction, so you can strike when they least expect it.

Creating and Breaking Patterns: Establish a predictable pattern of punches or movements. When your opponent starts reacting to "that regular ticking of the clock", break the pattern with something unexpected, completely catching them off guard. This method outsmarts your opponent and leads them into traps.

Observation and Adjustment

Throw a predictable series of punches, such as a jab-cross combination, and pay attention to where your opponent habitually moves their head to defend. Once you've identified their defensive response, repeat the same pattern, but break it by aiming your punch where their head has been dipping. This adjustment can catch them off guard and land a clean shot.

Unexpected Changes

Once you've recognized your opponent's reactions to your usual punches, don't just adjust your aim, use footwork and rhythm changes to catch them between defensive beats.

Breaking your movement pattern, stepping to a new angle, or pausing unexpectedly can throw off their timing and trigger an instinctive reaction that leaves them open.

This creates a devastating surprise attack and opens clean punching lanes where they least expect it.

I remember the first time I truly applied this in sparring. I had understood the concept, but seeing how effective it was in real time blew my mind. The moment I saw an opponent react exactly as I anticipated, and punished them for it, was like unlocking a new level in fighting.

One of the biggest fights where I consciously used these principles was against former world champion Tony Harrison, a slick, high-level technician who had already proven himself on the world stage. I was a major underdog, stepping up in weight, and most people gave me no shot. But under Roy Jones Jr.'s guidance, I relied on pattern breaks and deception to catch him off guard, wobbling him multiple times and landing more total punches and power punches overall. Even though my execution wasn't perfect and the fight ended in a controversial draw, it proved to me that these strategies work, even against a world-class opponent under the brightest lights.

Eyes as Deception: Direct Their Focus, Land Your Shot

Using your eyes to mislead your opponent can force them to defend the wrong area, creating openings for clean shots. By consistently looking at a specific target, such as the body before throwing a body shot, you condition them to expect an attack in that area. Once they start reacting to your gaze, you can break the pattern to land an unexpected strike up top.

Floyd Mayweather often used this tactic, glancing downward as if targeting the body before snapping a lead right hand to the head. This subtle misdirection made opponents brace for the wrong attack, leaving them exposed to precise, well-timed punches.

By controlling where your opponent focuses their defense, you dictate the exchanges. Looking down can draw their guard low, exposing their head for a well-placed shot. Looking up can make them raise their hands, opening their body for a devastating counter. This tactic isn't about waiting for an opening, it's about creating one on your own terms.

Predictability as a Weapon

The most devastating knockouts are from punches they don't see coming. Patterns can be created with any combination of punches, jabs, crosses, hooks and uppercuts. For instance, you might establish a pattern of throwing a double left jab followed by a right cross to the body. Watch for signs that your opponent has picked up on this. Do they start lowering their guard, anticipating the body shot? Are they timing a counter or shifting their weight to defend? Once you notice this, break the pattern by throwing a double left jab followed by an overhand right to the head, catching them completely off guard, as they were expecting another straight punch to the body.

Effective Patterns and Setups

These are just examples of how to build patterns and break them. The goal is to condition your opponent, then surprise them when they expect something familiar.

Jab-Body Hook Setup: Establish a pattern by jabbing to the body. Once your opponent starts reacting to the body jab, fake a jab to the body and come up with a lead hook to the head.

Body to Head Hook: Land two left hooks to the body. On the next one, fake low, then left uppercut to the head.

Jab-Hook-Back Hook to Uppercut Switch: Throw a jab, lead hook, and back hand hook combination a few times. Once your opponent starts expecting the same ending, switch the final hook into a rear uppercut. As they brace or dip to catch the hook, they drop right into your uppercut.

Key Tips for Patterns

Vary Your Patterns: Develop a wide array of sequences to keep your opponent guessing.

Train These Setups: Practice these sequences on the heavy bag, mitts, or with a sparring partner to develop muscle memory and the ability to recognize key openings in real time. Repetition sharpens instincts, when the moment comes, your body will react without hesitation.

Be Unpredictable: Break patterns at different points, sometimes on the first repetition, other times on the third or fourth.

Use Footwork: Include lateral movement, pivots and angles into your patterns for added deception.

Selling the Pattern

The key to making patterns effective is to convince your opponent that your next sequence of punches will be the same. Use similar body language and feints, and commit fully to your punches to make the pattern believable.

Tip: Add speed changes to pattern breaks. When it's time to break the pattern, hit the gas. Increase the speed of the pattern breaking punch, reducing the time between punches. Speeding up the disrupting punch makes it even harder to react to. That sudden burst of speed will catch your opponent completely off guard, leaving them wide open for the shot they won't see coming. This sharp change in tempo makes your pattern breaks even more dangerous and harder to defend against.

Practical Drills

- **Shadowboxing:** Practice your patterns during shadowboxing to make your sequences fluid and natural. Incorporate feints to simulate real fight conditions, disguising your speed changes and pattern breaks.
- **Heavy Bag Drills**: Work on your patterns with fluid, believable sequences on the heavy bag, focusing on power, speed variation, and precision.
- **Sparring**: Test your patterns in sparring to see how they work against a live opponent. Integrate feints and speed changes to further disrupt your opponent's timing and reactions.

Closing Thoughts

Setting up and breaking patterns is one of the most powerful tools you have as a fighter. It allows you to control the fight instead of just reacting. When you truly harness this skill, you can create your own openings, even against top opposition, and make them pay for their predictability. Remember: the most dangerous punches are the ones they never see coming.

Chapter 8
Strategies for Different Fighting Styles

"Box a fighter, and fight a boxer." [14]

Boxing isn't a one-size-fits-all sport. It's a complex game with many fighting styles. Every boxer brings their own unique approach to the ring. Some prefer to keep their distance and avoid punches, while others thrive by getting close and throwing fast combinations. To truly dominate in the ring, it's crucial to understand how different styles interact, and how to counter them with effective strategies. As the saying goes, "Box a fighter, and fight a boxer." This highlights the idea that every style or challenge your opponent presents has an answer. Recognizing it, adapting, and finding the right strategy is key.

There's also a common belief in boxing that 'styles make fights'. While styles can influence matchups, fights are rarely won on style alone. A counterpuncher isn't guaranteed success against an aggressive fighter, just as a pressure fighter doesn't automatically overwhelm a more passive opponent. What truly determines the outcome is the tactics and strategies you use. More importantly, it comes down to who has mastered themselves and their own style. Truthfully, a boxer can beat a fighter, and a fighter can beat a boxer. It all depends on who has fully developed their strengths, closed their gaps, and can impose their game when it matters most. The goal is to compete, but also to take control of the fight by exploiting your opponent's weaknesses and making their style work against them.

Although fighters may blend elements from different styles, they generally have a core style and particular tendencies that define

---

[14] Traditional boxing maxim. A fundamental strategic principle taught in boxing gyms worldwide, emphasizing the importance of adapting your style to counter your opponent's strengths.

their approach in the ring. Understanding this core style is key to identifying how to counter it effectively.

Common Boxing Styles

- Outside Boxer
- Pressure Fighter/In-Fighter
- Counter Puncher
- Volume Puncher
- Boxer-Puncher
- Brawler
- Southpaw
- Switch-Hitter
- Philly Shell/Shoulder Roll
- The Pure Boxer
- The Knock-Out Artist

Note: There are many variants of these styles, and each boxer is unique. However, for the sake of clarity, the above examples cover the universally known basic styles. These strategies are just options and generalized game plans. Always listen to your coach and develop what works best for you.

The upcoming examples of fighters in each category are divided into past and modern for reference. Over time, today's active fighters will become part of history, and new fighters will emerge who fit these styles. The goal of these examples is not to create a definitive list but to illustrate how different fighters have applied these styles at the highest level.

Overcoming the Distance: Defeating the Outside Boxer

Understanding the Outside Style

The outside boxer (or out-fighter) stays on the edge of their opponent's range, using quick movement, footwork, and long-range punches like jabs and crosses to maintain distance. Their goal is to control the ring while creating openings for counter-punches, keeping their opponents at bay while minimizing risk.

Outside boxers   often rely on reach, accuracy and ring generalship to avoid exchanges inside and frustrate opponents.

Some outside boxers focus purely on speed and footwork, while others patiently control distance with timing and minimal movement. Either way, their goal is to control space and keep the fight at their pace.

Key Characteristics

Movement and Positioning: Mastery of footwork keeps them at an optimal range, making it difficult for opponents to land clean punches.

Ring Generalship: They control space with movement, using footwork to stay off the ropes and avoid exchanges where they're most vulnerable.

Speed and Accuracy: They often focus on fast, precise punches that keep opponents at a distance, preventing inside exchanges.

Examples of Outside Boxers

Past: Muhammad Ali, Lennox Lewis, Thomas Hearns, Mark Breland, Cecilia Brækhus

Modern: Callum Smith, Luke Campbell, Chris Algieri, Erislandy Lara

Strategies to Face an Outside Boxer

Cut Off the Ring: Limit their movement by cutting off their angles and trapping them in corners or along the ropes. This forces them to fight on your terms, preventing them from using their footwork and range to escape exchanges.

Approach with Patience: Methodically close the distance while slipping or dodging their punches. A slow, calculated approach reduces risks and positions you for inside exchanges without rushing in recklessly. But that doesn't mean you have to be flat-footed, quick, explosive entries can be just as effective. You can close the distance fast, get your punches off, then pivot to the side and continue to fire, or disengage and reset outside their range. Smart pressure doesn't mean staying planted, it means knowing when to enter, when to stay, and when to exit.

Use Feints, Head Movement and Timing: Feints and head movement make it difficult for an outside boxer to time their jabs and counters. Vary your rhythm and attack patterns to disrupt their timing, forcing them to miscalculate and creating opportunities for you to attack. Combine this with an understanding of distance, with sharp timing and footwork, and you can break through an outside boxer's ability to maintain their preferred range.

Control Their Lead Hand: Parry or paw at their lead hand to disrupt their jab, which is their primary tool for maintaining distance. You can also simply counter their jab—time it and fire over or under it to take it away. Controlling their lead hand takes away their rhythm and opens up opportunities for you to close the gap and attack.

Safety Note: Keep your head off the centerline (left or right) when you parry or paw at the lead hand of a longer outside boxer, and keep the free hand ready to catch the cross/hook.

Bait Them In and Counter: You don't always have to apply pressure. Sometimes, using intelligent movement and light punches can lure them into closing the distance themselves. Another effective method is to throw a punch and close the distance as they fire back, slipping their counter and landing a well-timed punch of your own. This allows you to use their reaction to your advantage and close the gap.

Maintain Pressure: Apply steady, intelligent pressure to keep them from resetting. The goal is not only to move forward, it's to disrupt their rhythm, limit their escape routes, and force them into uncomfortable exchanges.

Rough Them Up Inside and Target the Body: Once you get inside, make it uncomfortable for them by staying close and roughing them up. Combine body shots with short hooks to sap their stamina and slow their movement. Body shots are particularly effective for wearing down an outside boxer who relies on mobility and endurance.

Use Angles and Stay Low: When closing the gap, stay compact and use angles (avoid straight-line entries) to make yourself a harder target. This keeps you elusive while positioning yourself to attack from better openings.

The Relentless Force: The Pressure Fighter/In-Fighter

Understanding the Pressure Fighter

Also known as swarmers or in-fighters, pressure fighters thrive on close-quarters combat. Their strategy revolves around overwhelming opponents with a constant barrage of attacks, making it difficult for their opponent to counter or defend effectively. Pressure fighters rely on relentless forward movement to trap their opponents, pushing them into a defensive position where they can wear them down with continuous pressure.

Because of this, it's strongly advised to develop skill and composure on the inside. Some pressure fighters will inevitably force you to fight in the pocket, whether you want to or not. Building comfort in this range is crucial, so that when you're crowded or tied up inside, you stay composed, pick your punches wisely, and maintain strong defensive awareness. This advice also applies when facing volume punchers or brawlers who can overwhelm you in close-range exchanges.

Key Characteristics

Aggressive Forward Movement: Pressure fighters relentlessly move forward, staying just within their opponent's punching range, forcing them to fight on the back foot.

High Energy and Stamina: This style requires incredible cardio, as the pressure fighter's goal is to exhaust the opponent over time with non-stop aggression.

Footwork and Positioning: Effective footwork is essential for maintaining pressure while avoiding counters. Pressure fighters aim to cut off the ring, controlling space and limiting their opponent's movement.

Close-Range Combat: They rely on head movement and short-range punches like hooks and uppercuts, constantly staying within striking distance to keep the fight at close quarters.

Body Attacks: Known for targeting the body, pressure fighters often operate under the principle "kill the body and the head will fall", wearing down their opponent's stamina and defenses over time.

Ring Control: Pressure fighters look to trap their opponents against the ropes or in corners, using the ring to limit their movement and create openings for sustained attacks.

Unlike brawlers, who rely on raw power and sometimes chaotic aggression, pressure fighters use calculated pressure to break down opponents systematically. They thrive on keeping their opponent uncomfortable and unable to establish an offensive rhythm. While they take risks by staying in the pocket, their ability to absorb punches and maintain a high work rate is critical to their success.

Not all pressure fighters overwhelm with volume, some apply mental pressure through presence, positioning, or patiently creeping forward. But the goal is the same: to make you uncomfortable and reactive.

Examples of Pressure Fighters

Past: Mike Tyson, Henry Armstrong, Julio Cesar Chavez, Antonio Margarito, Ricky Hatton, Christy Martin

Modern: Román González, Isaac "Pitbull" Cruz, Brandon Figueroa, Jaime Munguia, Gennady Golovkin

Strategies to Face a Pressure Fighter

Keep Calm Under Pressure: Pressure fighters want to overwhelm you mentally. To cause you to force decisions, provoke mistakes, and draw you into their fight. The key is mental discipline. Stay committed to your plan and don't fight emotionally. When they crowd your space, don't panic. A calm fighter thinks clearly, sees openings, and avoids costly mistakes. Some pressure fighters don't overwhelm with punches right away, they use presence alone to make you move unnecessarily, burning energy and making you easier to break down later. Don't fall for the trap. Stay relaxed and make every movement serve a purpose.

Move and Pivot: Use lateral movement and pivots to create angles that disrupt the pressure fighter's forward momentum. This makes it harder for them to land clean shots and forces them to reset their attacks.

Avoid Running: Don't give up too much ground by constantly backpedaling. Backing up excessively can encourage the pressure fighter and drain your energy while conserving theirs.

Exceed Their Volume: To beat a pressure fighter, sometimes you have to outwork them. Use consistent combinations and smart punch output to keep them reacting instead of dictating. If you control the exchanges, they struggle to build momentum. Mix lighter punches with power. You don't need to throw everything hard. What matters is keeping them occupied and working at a pace that challenges them without draining you.

Use Feints: Feints are a powerful tool against pressure fighters. They keep your opponent uncertain about when you're going to punch, which disrupts their rhythm and slows their forward momentum. Feints also allow you to read their reactions, especially when they're looking to step into range, helping you time their entries, pivot away, or meet them with a clean shot. Feints can force them to react instead of attack, giving you control over the tempo of the fight.

Exploit Openings: Pressure fighters can leave themselves open due to their aggressive nature. Capitalize on their mistakes with sharp, precise counterattacks. Well-timed counters can make them hesitate and disrupt their momentum.

Drain Their Stamina: Just as pressure fighters use body shots to wear down their opponents, you can use the same strategy to slow them down. Targeting the body can sap their energy and reduce their relentless pressure over the course of the fight.

Tip: Consistency with the lead hand and jab is critical against pressure fighters. Use a stiff jab to the body to interrupt their forward momentum and make them think twice before charging in. Jab high and low, use step-back counters, and pivot off to reset the distance and avoid any last second punches.

Throw Uppercuts and Check Hooks: Catch Them Coming In

Uppercuts: Use uppercuts to target their head or body as they move forward. Uppercuts are especially effective against pressure fighters who tend to lean in when closing the distance. You can also step back to create space before countering with an uppercut, or time them as they charge in, catching them mid-motion. Just be cautious, throwing an uppercut at the wrong time can leave you open to a hook or overhand. It's safest to launch when they're mid-step or committed to a missed punch.

Check Hooks: A check hook is a hook thrown as a counter to an aggressive opponent closing the distance. There are two ways to execute it:

1. **Step Back, Then Hook:** As they charge in, take a quick step back to create space, then throw the hook as they overcommit. This makes them walk right into the shot.

2. **Hook and Pivot Out:** Instead of stepping back, throw the hook while simultaneously pivoting to the side, using their momentum against them and creating an angle to escape.

Both variations are effective for disrupting their forward pressure, forcing them to reset, and keeping you in control of the exchanges.

Unpredictability: Avoid throwing full-power punches every time. Varying your power and tempo keeps the pressure fighter guessing, which throws off their timing and makes them hesitant to commit. The less predictable you are, the harder it becomes for them to anticipate your setups or brace for hard shots.

Manage Recovery: Pressure fighters look for signs that you're slowing down, especially after you throw a sequence of power shots. If you only throw hard, they'll read your fatigue and ramp up their attack when you're most vulnerable. Mixing in lighter punches allows you to stay active, conserve energy, and mask recovery periods, keeping them from capitalizing on your dips.

Cracking the Code: The Counterpuncher

Understanding the Counterpuncher

A counterpuncher thrives on making their opponents miss and then punishing them with well-timed punches. Instead of leading the action, they wait for openings by letting opponents get overly aggressive, then strike with precision. Counterpunchers use patience and sharp instincts to find the perfect moments to land their best shots.

Key Characteristics

Baiting and Timing: Counterpunchers use small movements and feints to lure opponents into throwing punches, then respond with quick, accurate counters.

Calm and Focused: They stay composed under pressure, making their opponents take risks, and then capitalizing on those mistakes.

Versatility: Counterpunching can work with many boxing styles, always focusing on making opponents miss and then making them pay.

Examples of Counterpunchers

Past: Juan Manuel Marquez, Jersey Joe Walcott, Laila Ali

Modern: Terence Crawford, Guillermo Rigondeaux, Canelo Alvarez, Jermell Charlo, Skye Nicolson

Strategies to Face a Counterpuncher

Use Feints to Break Their Rhythm: Feints can throw a counterpuncher off. By faking a punch, you can force them to react early, creating an opening for you to land clean punches when they're off-balance.

Bait and Time Their Counter: Throw punches to force a reaction, but don't just wait for their counter, use your punch as bait to draw it out, then time your own shot to land as they commit. This is a form of interception. Meeting their attack with yours. Do this with your head off the center-line, like slipping just outside a moving train while tossing your own strike down the track. As they throw their counterpunch, you fire your own shot at the same time, ideally from a slightly angled position, catching them mid-attack. This takes precision and confidence, but when executed correctly, it can have devastating effects. If you're centered, you're easier to hit, so angle off. By staying just off-line, you make yourself a harder target while still landing clean.

Change Your Pace and Increase Volume: Counterpunchers often prefer a slower, controlled pace where they can read and react to mistakes. Speeding up the fight with quick combinations can disrupt them, but the key is to mix up your rhythm, more than throw fast. Vary the speed of your punches, using quick bursts and slight hesitations to make them misread your timing. A higher punch volume also forces them to stay defensive and reduces their chances to find clean counterpunching opportunities.

Study Their Counters and "Attack Their Counter": Pay attention to how they react to your punches. Which shots do they like to counter, and what do they throw in response? Once you identify their pattern, use it against them. For example, if they always counter your jab, throw a jab to bait them, but this time, be a step ahead. Either slip, block, or pull back slightly to make them miss, then counter immediately. By anticipating their reactions, you take away their advantage and control the exchange.

Stay Mobile and Use Angles: Don't stand still or become predictable. Keep moving and change your angles of attack so they can't anticipate your next punch. Mix in subtle feints and direction changes, beyond just with your hands, but with your footwork.

Be Patient and Take Smart Risks: Don't rush or force punches. Be patient and look for the right moment to strike. When you do take a risk, make sure it's calculated and that you've found a gap in their defense.

Outpacing the Opponent: The Volume Puncher

Understanding the Volume Puncher Style

Volume punchers rely on a high punch output to overwhelm and wear down their opponents. Rather than focusing on power or precision, they maintain a steady barrage of punches to keep their opponents on the defensive. This constant pressure interrupts an opponent's flow, drains their energy, and creates opportunities for scoring through sheer work rate.

Key Characteristics

High Punch Output: Volume punchers throw a large number of punches per round to outwork and overwhelm their opponent.

Relentless Pressure: They apply constant physical and mental pressure, forcing their opponents to react and defend at all times.

Stamina and Endurance: Exceptional conditioning allows volume punchers to maintain a high work rate from start to finish.

Combination Punching: They rely on combinations rather than single punches, keeping their opponents off balance and unable to counter effectively.

Examples of Volume Punchers

Past: Joe Calzaghe, Paul Williams, Aaron Pryor, Henry Armstrong, Dmitry Pirog, Antonio Margarito, Christy Martin

Modern: Shawn Porter, Dmitry Bivol, Vasyl Lomachenko, Leo Santa Cruz, David Benavidez, Tiara Brown, Katie Taylor

Strategies to Face a Volume Puncher

Stay Mobile: Constant movement makes it difficult for volume punchers to set up their combinations. Stay light on your feet, moving in and out to avoid being a stationary target.

Lateral Movement and Feints: Incorporating side-to-side movement with feints forces volume punchers to adjust their timing. Feints can make them hesitate, creating openings for you to counter or move before they establish their pace.

Distance Management: Keep the fight at a distance where the volume puncher's output becomes less effective. Control the range. Use your jab to maintain control of the distance and prevent them from closing in and overwhelming you with combinations.

Break Their Flow: If they close the distance, tie them up or pivot out to stop their attack. Volume punchers thrive on rhythm. Disrupt it with smart footwork, angles, and well-placed counters before they can regain control.

Exploit the Gaps Mid-Attack: Whether it's a single counter or a flurry, volume punchers often leave split-second openings between punches. If you recognize their rhythm, you can slip a shot between their combinations and break their momentum.

Neutralize Their Combinations: Smother their punches by crowding them with inside positioning, making their shots ineffective. Use short, well-placed counters and strategic clinching to halt their momentum, force them to reset, and control the pace of the fight.

Control the Tempo: Don't allow the volume puncher to dictate the pace. Set a rhythm that works for you, and avoid getting drawn into high-tempo exchanges where they excel.

Vary Your Speed: Mix up the speed and intensity of your attacks. Changing the rhythm of your punches makes it harder for the volume puncher to anticipate your next move and adjust their approach.

The Versatile Fighter: The Boxer-Puncher

Understanding the Boxer-Puncher Style

Boxer-punchers combine the speed and skill of out-boxers with the power of brawlers. They possess strong jabs, counter-punching abilities, and better defense than brawlers, yet they pack a punch capable of ending fights. Unlike more defensively focused boxers, they are calculated in their approach, engaging aggressively when they see clear openings.

Key Characteristics

Hand Speed and Power: A combination of quick hands and knockout power.

Strong Jab and Counters: Effective jabs and counter-punching skills to keep opponents on edge.

Versatility: Capable of switching between defensive and aggressive styles, making them unpredictable.

Balanced Mobility: While not as elusive as pure defensive boxers, boxer-punchers can move well when needed. Many sit on their punches to generate power, but their ability to mix movement with offense makes them dangerous in both exchanges and counter-attacks.

Boxer-punchers are adaptable and can switch between different styles, making them a tough challenge for any opponent. Their unpredictability and ability to mix up tactics give them a significant advantage, though they may not always excel in one specific area compared to specialists.

Examples of Boxer-Punchers

Past: Sugar Ray Robinson, Roberto Duran, Sugar Ray Leonard, Roy Jones Jr., Alexis Argüello, Erik Morales, Lucia Rijker

Modern: Keith Thurman, Gervonta Davis, Teofimo Lopez, Naoya Inoue, Alycia Baumgardner, Claressa Shields

Strategies to Face a Boxer-Puncher

Identify Weaknesses: Analyze their habits to find and exploit weaknesses. Boxer-punchers may vary their approach, but they often have specific tendencies when committing to power punches or transitioning between offense and defense. Look for moments when they plant their feet to throw hard shots, or when they momentarily reset after countering, these are your openings. They may also have certain go-to counters or a preferred punch that carries the most power. Recognizing these patterns allows you to anticipate and neutralize their best weapons.

Disrupt Their Rhythm: Boxer-punchers thrive on setting traps and mixing power with defense. Use feints and change the pace of your attacks to throw them off balance and prevent them from getting comfortable.

Defensive Awareness: Boxer-punchers can deliver knockout power when exchanging shots with their opponents. Be cautious of their counter-punching ability and avoid getting drawn into firefights where they can capitalize on their strength.

Conditioning and Stamina: Some boxer-punchers are most dangerous in the middle rounds when they leverage both power and speed. By maintaining a consistent work rate and staying defensively responsible, you can take control as the fight progresses and their explosiveness becomes harder to sustain.

Use Angles and Movement: Employ lateral movement and angles to avoid their power punches and create opportunities for your own attacks. Boxer-punchers often plant their feet to generate power, which leaves them open to sharp angles and quick counters.

The Strategic Challenge: Overcoming the Southpaw

Understanding the Southpaw Style

Southpaws are generally left-handed fighters who lead with their right hand and right foot. Their stance and angles can be tricky for orthodox fighters to navigate, as most boxers are trained primarily against other orthodox fighters. This unique stance creates challenges in timing and distance, making it crucial to employ specific strategies when facing a southpaw.

Key Characteristics

Unconventional Angles: Southpaws create unfamiliar angles for punches, which often disrupt the defense of orthodox fighters, making it harder for them to anticipate attacks.

Footwork and Mobility: Southpaws use their footwork not only to find attacking angles, but also to maintain distance and evade counterattacks, making them harder to pin down.

Southpaw Power Shots: Southpaws often rely on powerful left-handed shots, using them as the primary tools to control the fight and push their opponent back.

Examples of Southpaws

Past: Pernell Whitaker, Sergio Martinez, Ronald "Winky" Wright, Manny Pacquiao, Michael Nunn, Guillermo Rigondeaux

Modern: Errol Spence Jr, Zab Judah, Jesse "Bam" Rodriguez, Amanda Serrano

Strategies to Face a Southpaw (For Orthodox Fighters)

Dominate the Lead Foot Game: The battle for lead foot positioning is crucial when facing a southpaw. While it's often advised to keep your lead foot outside of the southpaw's to gain superior angles, positioning your lead foot inside can also offer advantages depending on the situation.

- **Outside Lead Foot**: Moving your lead foot outside the southpaw's lead foot gives you a better angle to land your straight right and keeps you outside their powerful left hand.

- **Inside Lead Foot**: Stepping inside can create new angles for close-range attacks like body shots and hooks. This forces the southpaw to adjust and can disrupt their rhythm.

Movement Strategies: Understanding when and how to move against a southpaw is key to neutralizing their attacks. While circling left is traditionally taught to keep the lead foot outside, circling right can be just as strategic when done carefully.

- **Moving to Your Left (Outside Their Lead Foot)**: Circling left allows you to position your lead foot outside of theirs, reducing the effectiveness of their left hand while giving you better angles for your own attacks, especially your right cross or hook. This movement forces the southpaw to turn and reset, making it difficult for them to maintain control and creating openings before they can launch their left hand.

- **Moving to Your Right (Towards Their Back Hand)**: Moving to your right brings you into the path of the southpaw's strong left hand, but it can be used strategically. By anticipating their left hand and preparing a counter, you can catch them off-guard with a deadly punch, exploiting their opening as they commit to the power shot.

Lead Hand Dominance:

Establishing lead hand dominance is one of the most effective strategies against a southpaw. The goal is to control their jab hand to prevent them from setting up their attacks and limit their ability to land punches.

- **How It Works**: By constantly tapping, parrying, or pawing at their lead hand with your jab, you keep them occupied and disrupt their rhythm. This makes it harder for them to use their jab effectively, forcing them to readjust while giving you chances to land your own punches first.

- **Creating Openings**: Once you've established control over their lead hand, you can create openings for your right hand or hooks, dictating the pace of the fight and keeping them on the defensive. You can also parry their lead hand downward, then immediately follow with your own jab over the top, exploiting the opening. This can be combined with multiple jabs while moving outside of the opponent's lead foot, making it even harder for them to reset or respond.

Straight Right Hand:

The straight right hand is a great weapon against a southpaw. It can pierce their defense when thrown down the middle, exploiting the open angle between their guard.

- **Break Through Defense**: A clean, well-timed straight right can disrupt their positioning and throw them off balance, especially when you time it after slipping their jab.

- **Time It After Slipping Their Jab:** Many southpaws rely on their jab to set up their offense. If you slip it to the outside or inside, you create a perfect lane for your right hand down the middle.

Use Feints to Disrupt Their Rhythm: Southpaws thrive on timing and distance control, so using feints can throw them off balance and force them to react prematurely.

- **Feints as Setups**: Feints create hesitation, allowing you to capitalize on defensive reactions. This is a great setup for your right cross or a quick combination after drawing them out.

- **Analyze Defensive Patterns**: Test their reactions with simple punches to see where they instinctively move their head when avoiding strikes. Once you recognize their habit, use it against them, follow up with a shot aimed where they typically move, catching them off guard.

Strategies for Southpaws Facing Orthodox Fighters

Southpaws can apply the same strategies in reverse against orthodox opponents. The same battle for lead foot positioning, angles, and counter tactics apply—just flipped. The key remains controlling positioning, capitalizing on openings, and dictating the exchanges.

Southpaw vs Southpaw

When two southpaws face each other, the same principles apply as in an orthodox vs. orthodox matchup. Since both fighters share the same stance, the lead foot battle, angles and movement strategies become a mirror match. Instead of worrying about navigating an unorthodox stance, the focus shifts to who can control positioning and timing better. Just like an orthodox fighter would try to establish control over another orthodox fighter, a southpaw must apply these strategies against another left-hander to gain the upper hand.

The Unpredictable Opponent: The Switch-Hitter

Understanding the Switch-Hitter Style

Switch-hitters are fighters who can fluidly switch between orthodox and southpaw stances, making them unpredictable and hard to read. This ability lets them attack from different angles, keeping their opponents guessing throughout the fight.

Key Characteristics

Stance Switching: The ability to switch stances during a fight, which confuses opponents and creates new openings.

Versatility: Skilled in both orthodox and southpaw techniques, allowing them to adapt to different situations and take advantage of new opportunities.

Unpredictability: Beyond merely switching stances, but the timing, rhythm breaks, and unexpected angles they create, makes it difficult for opponents to develop a consistent strategy.

Examples of Switch-Hitters

Past: Marvin Hagler, Naseem Hamed

Modern: Terence Crawford, Jaron Ennis, Brandon Figueroa, Josh Taylor

Strategies to Face a Switch-Hitter

Analyze Tendencies: Watch when and why they switch stances. Look for patterns, like favoring certain punches and counters from each stance, and prepare to take advantage of those tendencies.

Identify Their More Natural or Preferred Stance: Not every switch-hitter is equally effective in both stances. Pay attention to which stance they seem more fluid and confident in. If they switch often but tend to rely on one stance more for their key attacks or defensive maneuvers, that's likely their natural or preferred stance. Recognizing this can help you anticipate their tendencies and adjust your strategy accordingly.

Stick to Your Game Plan: Don't let their switching throw you off your game. Stay disciplined and focus on executing your own strategy.

Create Openings: Stay light on your feet and use angles to your advantage. Quick footwork can help you catch them during a stance switch when they might leave openings.

Exploit Openings Mid-Switch: Switch-hitters may make mistakes when transitioning between stances. They might momentarily square up (exposing their centerline), lose balance, or hesitate before throwing. These are the moments to strike aggressively. You can also sometimes catch them in between an exchange, especially when they are switching stances mid-combination, because this becomes a habit for some fighters. If you time it right, you'll nail them while they're shifting and throwing at the same time. This is particularly dangerous for them because they're often completely square in that moment, while you're landing a flush shot.

Punish Hesitation: Some switch-hitters may use constant switching as a bluff to make opponents second-guess their attack. Don't let it freeze you. Attack when they hesitate or reset.

Develop Skills for Both Orthodox and Southpaw Opponents: Whether or not your opponent switches stances, you need to be comfortable fighting both styles. Knowing how to position yourself correctly, which counters work best, and how to defend against both stances will make you adaptable no matter what.

Train Against Switch-Hitters in Sparring: If you can, get live reps against fighters who actually switch stances. The more experience you get reacting to stance switches, the easier it will be to handle them in a real fight.

The Raging Bull: Anatomy of a Brawler

Understanding the Brawler

The brawler, or slugger, is all about raw power and relentless aggression. They thrive on overwhelming their opponents with relentless pressure and heavy punches. Brawlers are not concerned with finesse or defense as much as overpowering their opponent with brute strength and sheer volume. Brawlers excel in turning fights into slugfests, where their ability to absorb punishment and land powerful shots becomes their greatest weapon.

Key Characteristics

Power and Durability: Knockout power and an iron chin. Their ability to take damage and keep moving forward is often their greatest asset.

Aggressive Offense: Their goal is to smother opponents with pressure and powerful punches, forcing them into exchanges where the brawler can use their strength to dominate.

Relentless Pressure: Brawlers are relentless in their pursuit of their opponent, willing to trade shots and turn the fight into a physical war of attrition.

Examples of Brawlers

Past: Jack Dempsey, Ray Mancini, Marcos Maidana, Arturo Gatti, Ricardo Mayorga, Micky Ward, Ruslan Provodnikov

Modern: James Kirkland, Subriel Matias, Gabriel Rosado, Brandon Ríos, Emanuel Navarrete, Heather Hardy

Strategies to Face a Brawler

"The bull can't charge in a circle." [15]

Use Footwork and Movement: Good footwork is essential to neutralizing a brawler's power. Keep them turning by using pivots, lateral movement, and angles. This makes it difficult for them to plant their feet and generate power. Combine this with jabs and combinations to disrupt their rhythm and force them to reset.

Stay Composed and Keep Your Distance: Brawlers thrive on intimidation and close-range combat. Stay calm and stick to your game plan, using footwork and sharp shots to keep them at a distance. By maintaining range, you minimize their ability to use their power effectively.

---

[15] Traditional boxing maxim. A principle commonly taught in boxing gyms to emphasize the importance of lateral movement against aggressive opponents.

Use Feints, Counters, and Catch Them "In Between": Feints can disrupt the brawler's rhythm and make them commit to attacks prematurely. When they throw wide, looping punches, catch them "in between" by timing your shots precisely as they open up. Counterpunching during their attack is highly effective because they leave themselves vulnerable in these moments.

Draw Them Into Traps: Lure the brawler into overcommitting by using subtle pauses in your movement. Make them think you're open or hesitating, causing them to rush in. When they do, counter while they're off balance or mid-attack.

Mix Up Your Attacks: Don't rely on single punches. Use combinations to increase your chances of landing clean shots and to keep the brawler from resetting. Additionally, target the body to reduce their stamina and slow their relentless aggression.

Employ Clinching Techniques: When the brawler gets too close, initiate clinches to neutralize their power. Clinching helps prevent heavy blows and gives you the chance to reset the fight on your terms. (See Chapter 5 for more details on clinching.)

Philly Shell: Shoulder Roll Excellence

Understanding the Philly Shell Style

The Philly Shell, also known as the shoulder roll, is a defensive boxing technique focused on avoiding punches and setting up counters. Fighters using this style keep their lead hand low and their back hand high to protect both the chin and the front of the face, and they use the shoulder to block and deflect incoming punches. This style demands quick reflexes, good timing, and smart positioning.

Key Characteristics

Defensive Mastery: The shoulder roll allows fighters to use their shoulder to block punches while their back hand shields their chin and face from incoming strikes.

Counterpunching: Fighters using the shoulder roll excel at turning their opponents' mistakes into quick counterattacks.

Elusiveness: Small head movements and body shifts make them difficult to hit cleanly.

Examples of Shoulder Roll Practitioners

Past: George Benton, James Toney, Nicolino Locche

Modern: Floyd Mayweather Jr., Anthony Yarde, Caleb Plant, Tevin Farmer

Strategies to Beat the Philly Shell

Change Angles Fast: To break through the shoulder roll defense, you need to change your angle quickly when your opponent is planted. A fast pivot to the side can open up targets that the shoulder roll normally protects. Once you've moved, attack the new opening before they can reset.

Take Control: A strong and steady jab can mess up their rhythm, forcing them to react instead of taking charge of the fight. You can also jab and quickly turn it into a hook, since Philly Shell users often catch the jab with their rear hand, leaving them exposed to hooks wrapping around their guard.

Open Up Targets: Keep jabbing to both the body and head to keep them guessing and create chances to land bigger punches. Jabbing to the body followed by a cross to the head can be especially effective, since it draws their attention low and makes it harder to time or see the cross coming, disrupting their ability to shoulder roll the shot.

Break Down Their Defense: Punches to the shoulder, chest, and stomach can wear down a shoulder roll user, especially since these areas are less protected. Hitting the lead shoulder is especially effective since the hand is kept low in this defense. Striking the shoulder can disrupt their ability to block punches and set up follow-up shots to the head or body. Attacking these spots will eventually weaken their defense, making it easier to hit cleaner shots.

Predict Their Head Movement: Fighters using the shoulder roll often dip their heads to one side or the other to avoid punches. Instead of aiming at where their head is, throw to where it's going to be.

Body Shots: Attacking the ribs and stomach, especially by punching around the elbows, can slow them down and make it harder for them to avoid your punches. Targeting the sides of the body can expose vulnerabilities.

Drain Their Energy: Consistent body shots wear down their stamina, making them less mobile and less effective with their defense.

Change the Speed: Fighters using the shoulder roll rely on rhythm and anticipation. Mixing up the speed of your punches disrupts their timing and makes it harder for them to counter cleanly.

Surprise Them: Start with simple straight shots to probe their defense. Then suddenly shift to hooks or uppercuts when they're expecting another straight. This unpredictability breaks their pattern recognition.

Make Them React Too Soon: Shoulder roll users are often reactive. Feinting draws out their slips or rolls prematurely, giving you clean windows to strike.

Create Openings: Their defense relies on calm and calculated responses. Feints inject chaos. Use it to create gaps, then follow up before they reset.

The Pure Boxer: Finesse Over Force

Understanding the Pure Boxer Style

A pure boxer prioritizes skill, defense, and timing over aggression. Their focus is on landing clean punches while staying out of danger, using footwork and distance control to keep the fight on their terms. Rather than relying on power, pure boxers use sharp technique to stay ahead, maintaining range and taking advantage of their opponent's mistakes. They focus on hitting without getting hit, keeping themselves in control throughout the fight.

While they excel at range, some pure boxers are also highly capable at close quarters. Their technical ability, defensive awareness, and timing allow them to operate in the pocket without taking significant damage, proving that finesse and control can exist even on the inside.

Key Characteristics

Controlling the Fight: The jab is essential for pure boxers. It helps maintain distance, disrupts the opponent's rhythm, and sets up other punches. With the jab, they keep their opponent at bay, dictating the pace and direction of the fight.

Distance Management: Pure boxers excel at staying just out of reach while remaining ready to strike. They rely on efficient footwork to maintain the right range, using small adjustments to avoid punches and stay in a position to counter. They control the space with minimal effort, always poised to react.

Landing Clean Shots: Pure boxers don't generally throw a high volume of punches, instead focusing on landing effective, well-timed shots. They look for the right moment to strike, making each punch count while avoiding unnecessary exchanges.

Punishing Mistakes: Pure boxers are excellent at making their opponents miss, then quickly countering with well-placed shots. Their defense creates openings for counterattacks, turning their opponent's aggression against them as they become increasingly frustrated and make mistakes.

Controlled Engagements: Pure boxers minimize risk by engaging only when they see a clear opportunity. They don't rush into exchanges, preferring to wait for their opponent to make a mistake, allowing them to stay safe while outscoring their opponent.

Examples of Pure Boxers:

Past: Gene Tunney, Willie Pep, Muhammad Ali, Benny Leonard

Modern: Chris Bird, Paulie Malignaggi, Devin Haney, Shakur Stevenson, Billy Joe Saunders, Mikaela Mayer

Strategies to Face a Pure Boxer

Apply Pressure and Close the Distance: Pure boxers thrive when they can control the distance. To disrupt their plan, apply constant pressure and close the gap, forcing them into exchanges where they're less comfortable. Limit their movement and make it difficult for them to dictate the fight. If possible, trap them along the ropes or in the corners, where their movement is limited and they're more vulnerable to sustained offense.

Disrupt Their Rhythm and Outwork Them: Pure boxers prefer to control the tempo. By increasing your own punch output and mixing up your rhythm, you can force them out of their comfort zone. A higher volume of punches disrupts their timing and forces them into exchanges they try to avoid.

Target the Body: Pure boxers depend on their mobility to stay elusive. Body shots can slow them down, reducing their ability to move effectively. As they tire, more openings for combinations and headshots will emerge.

Be Physical and Force Exchanges: Pure boxers avoid physical, close-range engagements. By making the fight more scrappy—clinching, roughing them up, and forcing inside exchanges—you can take them out of their rhythm and force them into situations where they're less effective.

Force Riskier Punches: Landing early scoring punches can push a pure boxer to take more chances. Since they prefer staying ahead on points, they may feel pressured to respond quickly if they fall behind. After landing your punches, be prepared for their counterattack. This creates openings for you to counter their more aggressive attempts or catch them in exchanges they typically avoid.

The Knockout Artist: Understanding the Puncher Style

Punchers are fighters whose primary goal is to land a fight-ending shot. Unlike fighters who rely on high-volume combinations or finesse, punchers aim for one decisive blow that can change the course of a fight. Their approach revolves around maximizing the force of their punch, making them a constant threat no matter the round.

Key Characteristics

Tremendous Power: Punchers throw with significant force, and their punches often have the ability to cause major damage with just a single strike.

Efficiency: Rather than overwhelming their opponent with a high volume of punches, they generally focus on accuracy and timing to make every punch count.

Calculated Approach: Some punchers wait for the perfect opening to land their knockout blow, rather than aggressively pushing forward at all times.

Examples of Punchers

Past: George Foreman, Sonny Liston, Kelly Pavlik, Earnie Shavers, Tommy Hearns, Julian Jackson, Gerald McClellan, Ann Wolfe

Modern: Gervonta Davis, Deontay Wilder, Rolly Romero, Martin Bakole

Strategies to Face a Puncher

Use Your Feet to Control the Fight: Against a puncher, movement is your first line of defense. Don't stand still and give them a stationary target. Make them chase you. If they can't plant their feet, they can't fully launch their power. Use lateral footwork, quick pivots, and changes of angle to keep them off balance.

Neutralize Their Power Punch: Identify their most dangerous punch. Whether it's a powerful right cross or a crushing left hook. Work to take it away. By countering or making them miss their best shot via footwork or head movements, you reduce their confidence and force them to rely on other tools that may not be as effective.

Disrupt Their Timing: Punchers rely on perfect timing to land their power shots. By using head movement, footwork, and feints, you can break their rhythm, making it difficult for them to set up their punches. Varying the tempo of your attacks keeps them from getting comfortable.

Capitalize on Their Mistakes: Punchers tend to fully commit when they throw, which leaves them vulnerable if they miss. By slipping or parrying their punches, you can counter with clean, accurate shots. And just because they hit hard doesn't mean they aren't vulnerable themselves. If they overextend or leave themselves exposed, they can be hurt as well.

Stay Focused for the Entire Fight: A puncher's power is dangerous at any moment, so it's important to maintain focus throughout the entire bout. Even a brief lapse in concentration can give them the opening they need. Stay disciplined, avoid unnecessary risks, and never let your guard down.

Target Their Body: Punchers generate their power from their legs and core. By targeting the body with consistent punches, you can weaken their power base, slow them down, and make it harder for them to throw with full force.

Take Away Their Range: Punchers are often most dangerous at mid-to-long range, where they can generate full power behind their punches. However, not all punchers rely on distance. Some are just as effective at close range. For those who rely on distance, closing the gap and staying inside their range can smother their shots, reducing the impact of their punches. By crowding them, using clinches, or forcing them to fight on the inside, you can minimize the effectiveness of their biggest weapons. When dealing with a puncher who thrives up close, staying just outside their preferred range is key. Use lateral movement, and well-timed pivots to keep them from planting their feet and generating power. Tying them up in the clinch at the right moments can also disrupt their rhythm, forcing them to reset.

Identify Their Weaknesses: Every puncher has habits that can be exploited. If they repeatedly throw the same punch or drop their hands after certain movements, you can use these tendencies to set traps. For example, if they favor a big right hand, prepare to slip and counter with a well-placed hook or cross when they miss.

Mental Approach to Facing a Puncher

Remain Composed: Punchers often rely on intimidation. Staying calm and composed under pressure allows you to avoid making reckless mistakes. When you stay patient, it becomes harder for them to dictate the fight.

Fight with Intelligence: Avoid unnecessary brawls. Stick to smart, technical boxing, using defense to wear them down.

Be Confident and Patient: Trust in your strategy and stay patient. Control the fight, don't let them rush you into exchanges, and instead, force them to make mistakes you can capitalize on.

Real-World Application: Breaking Down a Difficult Style

I once faced a fighter named Patrick Boozer. He was an experienced southpaw who used the Philly Shell defense and liked to build pressure as the rounds went on. He had never been stopped before, and he was known for pulling off upsets against undefeated prospects. I knew going in that it wasn't just about landing more punches; it was about landing the right ones at the right time, without giving away anything in return.

From the opening bell, I stayed disciplined. I focused on pacing, angles, and carefully chosen counters. I used the jab to go up and down, and made sure to touch the body early. No wasted movement. No unnecessary risks. I broke him down piece by piece from the outside, staying defensively responsible while finding small cracks in his shell. When the moment came, I recognized it. One of my shots visibly hurt him. That was the green light. I pressed, stayed composed, and closed the show.

It wasn't about fighting harder. It was about fighting smarter. That's how you deal with layered, tricky opponents: not with brute force, but with strategy, patience, and execution.

Chapter 9
Build the Style That Works for You

"When I was a child, every day, I would come home and watch every legendary champion. Every champion. Larry Holmes. Sugar Ray Leonard. Marvin Hagler. Mike Tyson. Roberto Duran. Julio Cesar Chavez. I mean this list goes on and on. There wasn't one fighter I wanted to be like. Some days I wanted to fight like Leonard. But then I wanted to have a style like Tommy Hearns. But then I wanted to be a killer like Mike Tyson. And when I took all those different champions, I said I'm gonna take a little bit from every one of them, and put it in one box, and see what we come up with." [16]—Floyd Mayweather Jr.

The Fighter's Identity

Who are you in that ring when no one's telling you what to do?

Every fighter eventually has to answer that for themselves.

Style isn't something you always set out to create. For some, it comes naturally through training. For others, it's shaped by a coach's system, the influence of fighters they admire, or the environment they train in. You may not even notice it happening at first. At first, you're just mimicking someone you admire. Then one day, you move in a way that just feels right.

What you're building is your identity in the ring. Not someone else's. It might borrow pieces from the fighters you respect, but the rhythm, the posture, the intention behind each shot becomes your own. There's no perfect formula. Just repetition, influence, and feel. And over time, it all begins to merge.

Build solid fundamentals, sprinkle in creativity.

Before you start getting too creative, make sure you've built a rock-solid foundation in the fundamentals. Creativity only works when it's grounded in sound technique. Always return to

---

[16] Mayweather Jr., Floyd. Interview from "30 Days in May" documentary, Showtime Sports, 2012.

the fundamentals as your base. That's your anchor. Then, build from there into your own rhythm, flow, and individuality.

Just be cautious not to confuse individuality with something that's actually a glaring weakness or flaw. Having your chin way in the air, or constantly getting hit because your hands are down, isn't style. It's a liability. Know the difference.

Developing your skills is paramount to becoming a successful fighter. While I won't dive into specific techniques, since many different styles can lead to success, I will stress the importance of finding what works best for you. Whether you bounce on your toes for mobility, stay flat-footed for power, or use a hybrid approach, the key is consistency and continuous refinement. Some fighters keep their hands high for defense, while others lower them for enhanced upper-body movement and unpredictability. Through practice and perseverance, you'll discover the style that suits you best.

And while the final style should feel like yours, don't underestimate the role of an excellent coach in shaping it. The right mentor helps you discover what works best for you, not by forcing a style, but by guiding you toward your strengths, tightening your weaknesses, and showing you what you may not see yet.

Trust your coach, but don't be afraid to explore within the system they give you. The best fighters are built through communication, trust, and shared vision.

Finding Your Style

Every fighter has a unique style that plays to their strengths. Some prefer a quick-footed, mobile approach, bouncing on their toes to control distance and avoid attacks. This style relies on speed, reflexes and defensive skills to frustrate opponents and set up counterattacks.

Others favor a more grounded, flat-footed stance, staying planted to generate powerful punches while maintaining a solid frame. This approach emphasizes strength, durability and timing, wearing down opponents and landing heavy blows.

Many fighters find success with a hybrid approach, blending mobility with power. They switch between quick movement to evade and counter, and then plant their feet to deliver devastating strikes when the moment is right.

Each style can be effective, and the best choice depends on your physical attributes, skills and preferences. The key is to select a style that highlights your strengths while covering your weaknesses.

By this point, you've learned key skills like footwork, movement, and punch variation, the backbone of any successful fighter. Now it's time to combine them into a style that fits you.

Understanding Different Styles

To develop your own style, it helps to first get familiar with the different established styles in boxing we explored in the previous chapter. Whether it's the out-boxer, pressure fighter, or counter-puncher, each comes with its own strengths and weaknesses. By studying these styles, you can find elements that suit your natural abilities and decide what to add to your game.

This is where you move beyond the basics and start experimenting with different ways to move, defend and attack.

Understanding these styles gives you a broader palette to work with as you paint your own masterpiece in the ring.

Study the Greats: Learning from Legends

Immerse yourself in the study of great boxers. Watch and analyze their footwork, punch combinations, defensive tactics and counter-punching techniques. This in-depth study provides valuable insights into how these techniques can be integrated into your own style.

While there's a lot to learn from the greats, your goal isn't to copy them move for move. Instead, take what works for you and shape it to match your own strengths and abilities. Just as Floyd Mayweather Jr. did with his idols.

For example, Mike Tyson's "slip and rip" technique was one of the most devastating counterattacks in boxing. He would slip just outside an opponent's punch, staying within striking range, then explode with a vicious hook or uppercut before they could recover. His ability to turn defense into immediate offense made him one of the most feared punchers in history. Studying this kind of technique teaches you how to punish openings rather than just avoiding punches.

Experimentation and Adaptation: Finding What Fits

Creating your style takes trial and error. You'll try techniques from different fighters. Some will click, and others won't, and that's completely normal. The important thing is to stay open to experimenting and adjust as you figure out what works best for you.

As you go through this process, you'll start honing your approach, finding the moves that feel the most natural and effective. Over time, these techniques will become second nature, giving you the confidence to fight with your own unique flair.

Training Tips

- **Experiment:** Try different stances and movements during training to discover what feels natural and enhances your strengths.

- **Consistency**: Once you find what works, drill it consistently to refine your skills and make your style second nature.

- **Adaptation:** Stay open to adjustments as you gain more experience and face different opponents. Being able to adapt is often what defines high-level fighters and allows them to stay one step ahead.

Customization: Making It Your Own

As you experiment and gain experience, you'll start to notice which techniques and strategies feel right for you. This is when you can begin tailoring your style, mixing different elements to play to your strengths and cover your weaknesses.

Customizing your style is an ongoing process. It takes dedication, practice, and the flexibility to keep evolving as you grow as a fighter. With every fight and training session, your style will sharpen, becoming more effective and natural over time.

Continuous Improvement: The Never-Ending Journey

Developing your style is not a one-time effort but a continuous journey. It demands relentless dedication, constant practice, and ongoing experimentation. By watching other fighters, trying out new techniques, and adjusting your style to match your strengths, you'll stay sharp and ahead of the game. As you grow, so will your style, keeping you fluid and hard to predict. Each fight and training session is a chance to fine-tune your approach, letting your individuality show in the ring as you climb through the ranks. The greats never stopped refining. Neither should you. Let your style develop, but never forget what built it.

Chapter 10
Switch-Hitting:
The Power of Ambidexterity in Boxing

"You should not have a favorite weapon, nor likes and dislikes."[17]
—Miyamoto Musashi, The Book of Five Rings

Switch-hitting, the ability to fluidly switch between orthodox and southpaw stances, is a deadly weapon in boxing. It can keep opponents confused, break their rhythm, and create new openings. Fighters like Terrence 'Bud' Crawford, Marvin Hagler, and Jaron 'Boots' Ennis have used this skill to dominate, controlling fights by attacking from all angles. In this chapter, we'll dive into why this skill is such a game-changer.

Why Switch-Hitting Gives You the Upper Hand

Adapt on the Fly

When you can switch between stances, your opponent never knows what's coming. You'll be able to throw punches from angles they aren't used to defending, which forces them to reset and adjust. This keeps you in control, leaving them struggling to keep up. As they work to adjust to your changing angles, they also need to re-evaluate your habits and tendencies, making it harder for them to mount an effective offense while you're already launching your own attacks.

It can also help when facing a pressure fighter, as being able to fight from both stances makes it easier to move back, laterally, and still be ready to fire without being cut off or put in a

---

[17] Musashi, Miyamoto. "The Book of Five Rings" (Go Rin no Sho), circa 1645. Translated by Victor Harris, Overlook Press, 1974.

compromised position. For example, as the pressure fighter advances, you can step your front foot backward into a new stance. This not only shifts your angle but also brings your new lead hand closer, creating immediate openings for check hooks, jabs, or other quick punch variants before they can reset their position.

Continue the Assault

Switching stances lets you keep the pressure on without losing momentum. Instead of resetting after each attack, you stay active, catching your opponent from unexpected angles and keeping them on the defensive. The ability to flow seamlessly between stances makes it difficult for them to adjust, as they scramble to defend punches from positions they're not used to. This is especially effective when *shifting*—moving forward while transitioning to another stance, all while maintaining offensive momentum.

It can also help when cutting off the ring, as it takes away the opponent's escape routes and can put them directly in line with your power shot from the new stance.

Create New Openings

Switch-hitting doesn't just help maintain pressure, it literally forces your opponent to react to new threats. Each stance presents different attacking angles and exposes unique defensive gaps. For example, if your opponent tends to drop their rear hand when facing an orthodox jab, switching to southpaw could open the lane for a rear-hand left hook, which gives the shot more power and making it harder to anticipate than a lead hook from orthodox. If they already have trouble defending shots from that side, switching stances might let you target their blind spot more effectively.

Some openings only appear when viewed from a different stance. A stance switch can shift the dynamic, making weaknesses more pronounced or forcing an opponent into unfamiliar defensive adjustments. The ability to change the angle of attack in an instant keeps them from settling into a rhythm, increasing your chances of landing clean shots.

Elevate Your Dominant Side by Training the Other

Neural Adaptations: Training your non-dominant stance (meaning the side you don't naturally favor) strengthens the neural pathways in the brain. This enhances coordination and control on both sides, meaning your dominant side can become sharper, more fluid, and more precise as a result.

Increased Reaction Time & Cognitive Processing: Switching between stances forces your brain to process movements at a higher level. This increases reaction speed, fight IQ, and adaptability—even when you return to your dominant stance. The constant adjustments train your mind to make faster decisions in the ring.

Why Training the Weak Side Boosts Both: Most fighters have a noticeable difference in power between their dominant and non-dominant hands. Training your weaker side not only improves its effectiveness but also increases force production on your dominant side. This happens because the brain strengthens movement patterns and muscle recruitment, leading to overall stronger, more explosive punches.

Boxing Legends Who Perfected Switch-Hitting

Terence 'Bud' Crawford: Known for his ability to switch stances effortlessly, Crawford confuses and overwhelms opponents with his adaptability, constantly finding new openings to exploit.

Marvin Hagler: One of the toughest fighters in history, Hagler mastered the art of switch-hitting. This versatility combined with relentless aggression made him one of the most feared fighters in boxing.

Jaron 'Boots' Ennis: A unified welterweight world champion, Jaron Ennis can seamlessly fight from each side, combining speed and power from both stances, making him a force in the welterweight division. His unpredictability makes him a nightmare to prepare for.

The Tough Part: Defense in Both Stances

Switch-hitting is not purely about offense. You need to be just as sharp defensively in both stances. This means drilling your defensive moves in your non-dominant stance until you're just as comfortable protecting yourself, whether you're in orthodox or southpaw. It takes time, but the payoff is huge.

How to Train Your Switch-Hitting

Jab Practice: Dedicate one round to throwing jabs only from the orthodox stance, focusing on form and accuracy. In the next round, switch to southpaw and throw only jabs from that stance. This helps build muscle memory in both stances.

Footwork and Defense: Shadowbox while switching stances, practicing defensive movements like slipping, ducking, and blocking. Focus on how your defense changes in each stance, staying light on your feet while maintaining balance. To build comfort and adaptability, dedicate full rounds to each stance before incorporating stance switches into your movement.

Power Transitions: Switch stances while hitting the heavy bag, throwing combinations from both sides. Focus on maintaining power and control in both orthodox and southpaw to ensure fluidity in your transitions.

Defense from Each Stance: Partner with a training buddy to practice defensive drills. Take turns throwing light punches from both orthodox and southpaw stances while the other person defends in each stance. This helps you get comfortable defending from your non-dominant side.

Chapter 11
Adaptability: The Key to Becoming Unstoppable

"I have never won big fights just doing one thing, being one-dimensional." [18]—Andre Ward

In this game, adaptability is king. The ability to change and adjust during a fight can be the difference between winning and losing. A world-class fighter must shape themselves into whatever is needed to overcome their opponent. This chapter explores why being adaptable is so important and how developing this ability will take you to the next level.

The Essence of Adaptability

Adaptability in boxing isn't about having a fixed set of backup plans. It's about finding solutions in the moment. It's recognizing when something isn't working and making the necessary adjustments, whether that means changing your punch selection, altering your range, or shifting your overall approach to the fight.

If your opponent isn't biting on your feints, add more commitment or disguise them better. If they're timing your jab, double it up or mix in a lead hook to break their rhythm. If fighting on the outside isn't working, step in, rough them up and make it ugly. The best fighters don't just impose their game, they adjust, adapt and take control no matter how the fight unfolds.

---

[18] Ward, Andre. HBO Boxing post-fight interview following victory over Sergey Kovalev, June 2017. Ward discussing his multi-faceted approach to boxing strategy.

Why Adaptability Matters

"A true champion can adapt to anything." [19] —Floyd Mayweather Jr.

No two fights are alike. Opponents come with different strengths, weaknesses, and strategies. Being able to adapt quickly is key for a few reasons:

Handling Surprises: No matter how much you prepare, a fight may throw unexpected challenges at you. Your opponent might have a different style or use new tactics. Adaptability lets you handle these surprises effectively.

Exploiting Weaknesses: As the fight progresses, you may notice weaknesses in your opponent that weren't obvious before. Whether due to their fatigue setting in or the increased data you've gathered on their tendencies, adjusting your strategy to exploit these weaknesses can turn the fight in your favor.

Energy Management: The pace of a fight can change. Being able to adjust your tempo and conserve energy when needed helps ensure you're still strong in the later rounds.

Developing Adaptability

"Improvise, Adapt, and Overcome." [20]

Adaptability is not something you're born with, it's a skill that must be developed. Versatility is the key to adaptability. Having a diverse array of skills gives you the ability to find adjustments and other moves that will turn the tide back in your favor. Here are some ways to improve your adaptability:

Versatile Training: Train in various styles and techniques. Spar with different types of fighters—aggressive,

---

[19] Mayweather Jr., Floyd. From pre-fight press conference before Manny Pacquiao bout, March 2015. Often repeated throughout his career when discussing his adaptability in the ring.

[20] Traditional maxim popularized by the United States Marine Corps, widely adopted across disciplines including combat sports.

defensive, tall, short. This helps prepare you for any situation in the ring.

Film Study: Study your opponents carefully, but also review your own fights. When possible, watch your opponents fight live to catch nuances that might not be as clear on film, things like their energy shifts, reactions under pressure, and tendencies in real time. Analyze what strategies worked against them and where they showed weaknesses. At the same time, review your own fights to see what worked, what didn't, and why. This reflection helps you make the necessary adjustments to sharpen your approach.

Mental Flexibility: Develop a mindset that's open to change. Practice visualization where you imagine different fight scenarios and how you would adapt. This mental preparation primes you for making adjustments during a fight. For more on visualization and how to make it work for you, see Chapter 15.

Feedback and Reflection: After each fight, take the time to reflect on your performance. Seek feedback from your coach and sparring partners. Understanding where you can improve helps you become more adaptable in future bouts. Consider tracking key takeaways, whether by reviewing film, keeping notes on adjustments needed, or logging insights from your coach. Seeing patterns over time helps solidify improvements and sharpen your overall fight IQ.

In-Fight Adjustments

A good fighter can make adjustments fight by fight, a great fighter can make adjustments round by round.

The ability to make quick adjustments during a fight is what sets outstanding fighters apart. Some fighters need an entire training camp to make an adjustment, while great fighters adapt between rounds, even mid-exchange. They recognize when a strategy isn't working and tweak their approach on the spot.

- If your opponent keeps countering your jab, you don't wait until the next fight to fix it, you double it up, feint before throwing, or feint to bait their counter and punish them for it.

- If they're walking you down and smothering your shots, you adjust your distance, use lateral movement, or start countering inside to make them pay for their aggression.

- If your game plan was to box on the outside, but they're cutting off the ring effectively, you shift tactics—tie them up, pivot out at angles, or force them to reset before attacking.

Here's how you can apply this in the ring:

Stay Calm and Focused: Panicking will cloud your judgment. Keep your shoulders loose, reset your breath between bursts, and stay dialed in. Your ability to adapt relies on a clear mind.

Listen to Your Corner: Your coach sees things you might miss. Trust their guidance and be willing to change your approach based on their advice.

Small Changes: Minor adjustments can make a big difference. Tweaking your footwork, adjusting your guard, or switching up your punch combinations can disrupt your opponent.

Confidence in Change: Trust your ability to adapt. Confidence is essential for making changes work during a fight.

Practical Adaptation Techniques

In a fight, you might need to shift from being stationary and aggressive to moving your feet, creating angles, and "sticking and moving" to outmaneuver your opponent. On the other hand, you may need to switch from this mobile approach to using a high guard and "walking down" your opponent, closing the distance to apply pressure and land strong punches up close.

The Importance of Adaptability

"It's survival of the fittest, and the fittest are the ones who are highly adaptive." [21]

Adaptability is about thriving in the ring; no matter what. It's about becoming whatever you need to be and doing what it takes to win. Develop adaptability, and you'll be ready for any challenge. The ability to make key adjustments is crucial—It's what elevates fighters from being skilled to becoming truly exceptional.

---

[21] Adapted from Darwin's theory of natural selection, "On the Origin of Species" (1859). The concept of "survival of the fittest" was actually originally coined by Herbert Spencer in "Principles of Biology" (1864).

Chapter 12
Seize Control: Dominate Every Exchange

"Control the distance, control the fight." [22]
—Boxing maxim

In boxing, the one who dictates the terms isn't always the one throwing the most punches, it's the one pulling the strings. Techniques like frames, posts, pins, peels and the long guard allow you to dictate every exchange, turning defense into offense. When these tools are used together, they keep you in command, forcing your opponent to fight on your terms.

The Long Guard: Manage Distance and Set Traps

The long guard uses an extended lead hand to maintain distance and force your opponent to fight from the outside. It disrupts their rhythm and limits their ability to land clean punches. Hooks glance off your arm like a natural block.

It's a tool best suited for longer-range fighters, but with the right adjustments, even shorter fighters can use it in bursts to manage space and create opportunities to close the gap. It can also help pick off your opponent's long-range punches, as the extended hand can disrupt the path of incoming shots , another reason it can be effective for shorter fighters.

The **step-back** is absolutely essential, remaining stationary leaves you vulnerable to shots around your extended arms. Stepping back makes their attacks fall short, leaving them off-balance and open to counters. Tyson Fury uses the long guard to frustrate opponents, keeping them at range and punishing them with counters. Gervonta Davis, while not a traditional long-

---

[22] Controlling distance is one of the core tactical principles in boxing. Fighters who master range can dictate the pace, shut down opponents' strengths, and create openings for their own offense. This concept is central to the styles of great defensive boxers like Floyd Mayweather Jr., Vasiliy Lomachenko, and Pernell Whitaker.

guard fighter, tactically uses an extended lead hand against orthodox opponents to control their jab hand, especially against taller fighters, creating windows to slip inside and land explosive shots.

How to Train with the Long Guard

For Taller Fighters: Practice jabbing from the long guard and transitioning into power punches as your opponent steps within range. This position also places your glove closer to their face, making it harder for them to see punches coming.

For Shorter Fighters: Use the long guard momentarily to disrupt your opponent's jab and create hesitation—then slip inside and attack. After landing punches, extend your lead hand again to create a brief pocket of space and reset the exchange.

In Sparring: Use the long guard to control the tempo, forcing opponents to overreach and miss.

Posts: Track the Head and Disrupt Forward Aggression

A post extends your lead hand to your opponent's head or neck, halting their forward movement. Posts work naturally with the long guard, tracking your opponent's head to control their movement. This makes it difficult for them to launch effective forward aggression, forcing them to reset or attempt awkward punches.

By maintaining contact with their head, the post allows you to limit their angles of attack and guide their movement. Stepping back as you post makes it even harder for your opponent to close the gap, disrupting their rhythm and leaving them open for counters.

You can also use the post to briefly block their vision, creating confusion. Tommy Hearns used this technique against Jose 'Pipino' Cuevas, momentarily blinding him before landing a clean right hand that ended the fight. Posts must be quick, holding too long will draw a warning from the referee.

Posts frustrate aggressive fighters, forcing them to overreach. Muhammad Ali and Lennox Lewis used posts to track opponents and set up counters as they missed their punches.

Frames: Control Space and Limit Offense

A frame is a versatile tool for controlling close quarters and preventing your opponent's advance. Placing your forearm across their chest, shoulder, or near the side of their neck gives you the space to reset or attack. You can frame with your lead arm to line up clean shots with your rear hand, or frame with your rear hand to open up powerful attacks from your lead side. Floyd Mayweather Jr. used frames masterfully as part of his Philly Shell defense, especially in close-range exchanges. His frames created space and more importantly, reduced his opponent's offense, allowing him to escape tight situations or counter effectively.

Pins and Peels: Trap Hands and Open Angles

Frames can also act as pins, locking your opponent's upper body and exposing the sides of their head and body for hooks or uppercuts. With their movement restricted, you force them to fight on your terms, giving you control over tight exchanges. Canelo Alvarez excels at pinning his opponents, trapping their hands to create space for uppercuts and body punches.

On the inside, Roberto Duran was known for his mastery of pinning, using subtle traps to neutralize his opponent's offense and create openings for uppercuts and short hooks. After pinning their glove, you can peel it down to expose new openings. A quick peel creates immediate angles for hooks or crosses, breaking through even the tightest guard. One effective way to disguise the peel is to first occupy them with punches up top—get them covering up—then slip the peel in mid-combination when their focus is elsewhere. Vasiliy Lomachenko and David Benavidez use peels to create space and fire precise combinations inside.

Bringing It All Together: Mastering Control

Mastering frames, posts, pins, peels, and the long guard gives you the ability to dominate every exchange. Each tool builds on the others, turning defense into offense and keeping you one step ahead of your opponent. When used together, these techniques limit your opponent's offense, create openings, and allow you to control the fight's pace.

How to Combine These Techniques in Training

1. **Start with the Long Guard**: Use it to keep your opponent at bay and force them to overreach.

2. **Post to Track the Head and Limit Forward Aggression**: Use your post to track their movement and briefly block their vision, setting up a clean cross.

3. **Frame to Control Space and Limit Offense**: When on the inside, use your forearm to frame across their chest, shoulder, or neck, creating space to attack or reset.

4. **Pin and Peel to Open Shots**: Trap their glove with a pin, then peel it down to expose openings for hooks or body shots.

5. **Pivot to Create Angles**: After peeling, step aside to create an angle for your next shot.

With practice, these techniques will become second nature, allowing you to stay in control of every exchange. Mastering them ensures that you'll dictate the fight, always on your terms.

Chapter 13
The Importance of Studying Your Opponent

"Every fighter has a style and a strategy, and it's my job as a trainer to analyze and exploit weaknesses." [23]
—Emanuel Steward, Hall of Fame trainer

Understanding your opponent is one of the keys to success in the ring. The better you know their patterns and habits, the more prepared you'll be to react and take control.

Studying an opponent can be done in multiple ways, through film, live observation (if possible), and by analyzing their past performances against fighters with styles similar to yours. While it's important to study your opponent, your coach and team can also take on much of this responsibility, breaking down key tendencies and creating a game plan. This frees you up to focus on executing strategies rather than overanalyzing every detail yourself.

True preparation goes beyond watching a few fights: it's about being ready for anything they bring to the table. Beating your opponent is more than your physical ability, it's about understanding how they fight.

Deciphering Your Opponent's Boxing Style

Every opponent is different, and no single strategy works for everyone. To gain the upper hand, you need to learn how they operate in the ring.

Studying your opponent isn't about knowing their flashy moves or knockout highlights; it's about recognizing patterns, habits, and how they handle pressure. Do they come out strong and

---

[23]Steward, Emanuel. Quote from boxing training interview, ESPN Boxing, circa 2010. Steward was a Hall of Fame trainer known for his work at Kronk Gym and training numerous world champions including Tommy Hearns and Lennox Lewis.

aggressive, or do they take their time and build momentum? Are they defensive, waiting to counter, or do they prefer to take the lead and initiate exchanges? These details can guide your approach to the fight.

As we discussed in Chapter 8: Strategies for Different Fighting Styles, where we analyzed the various styles of fighting and strategies to overcome them, the key to success lies in recognizing how each style works and adapting your game plan accordingly. Whether you're facing a southpaw, a brawler, or a counter-puncher, your ability to decipher their movements and anticipate their next steps is vital.

This knowledge will help you neutralize their strengths and enable you to capitalize on their weaknesses, giving you the strategic edge in the ring.

It's also helpful to see how they've performed against fighters who have a style similar to yours. This can give you insight into how they might handle your approach and reveal any weaknesses in their game plan. Knowing how your opponent reacts gives you an advantage before the first bell even rings.

Fighters like Floyd Mayweather Jr. take this preparation to another level. He doesn't just study film, he looks into his opponent's lifestyle. Mayweather wants to know what his opponent eats, how they train, and even what they do outside the gym. This information can reveal weaknesses, like poor discipline or bad habits, that can be exploited in the ring. This level of preparation gives you an edge even before the fight begins.

Freddie Roach rose to legendary status as a coach by mastering the art of opponent analysis. His sharp observational skills and deep understanding of boxing allowed him to transition from fighter to one of the sport's greatest trainers. He meticulously studied his fighters' opponents, breaking down their tendencies and weaknesses, then structured sparring sessions and strategic game plans to exploit those patterns. This methodical approach gave his fighters a tactical edge and also cemented his reputation as a mastermind in the sport of boxing.

To get the most out of studying your opponent, pay attention to their tendencies:

- Do they move forward aggressively, or do they back off when under pressure?

- Do they initiate exchanges, or do they wait to counter?

- Do they favor a particular punch over the others?

- What combinations do they throw, and how do they react after finishing them?

- Do they slow down as the round progresses, or do they keep a steady pace?

- Do they use feints to trick opponents, or are their attacks more straightforward?

- How do they react when they're tired?

Recognizing these patterns gives you a tactical advantage. If you can predict their responses, you can plan your counters and time your shots more effectively.

Mastering Film Study for Boxing

> *"I needed to study his style. I needed to know all I could about him. Suddenly, watching the films one day, I saw what I had been hoping to find—he liked to throw a right hand to the body, and when he did, his jaw was open for my left hook."* [24]—
> Sugar Ray Robinson

A structured and detailed approach to film study can reveal patterns in your opponent's tendencies, giving you a strategic edge. Watching footage of your opponent allows you to analyze their strengths and weaknesses, but the key is to look beyond the obvious. It's about finding patterns, how they move, how they position themselves, and how they react under pressure. This analysis is not only useful for fight night, it should also

---

[24] Sugar Ray Robinson, describing his fight-planning process before his May 1, 1957 rematch with Gene Fullmer, Chicago Stadium—recounted in *Sports Illustrated*, "A Punch for History," May 13, 1957, and in fight archives of 3Kings Boxing.

guide your training leading up to the fight. You can structure your sparring to mimic your opponent's tendencies, drilling the most effective counters, and use shadowboxing and mitt work to reinforce strategies that will work against them.

Effective Film Study Techniques

Slow It Down: Watching fight footage at slower speeds —like 75% or even 50%—can help you catch small details, like footwork, hand placement, and defensive reactions that might be missed at full speed. UFC champion Georges St-Pierre revealed that he used this technique during his preparation to gather valuable insights he could exploit in his fights.

Watch Multiple Fights: Don't just watch one fight, see how your opponent handles different types of fighters. Look for habits that show up in every match. These tendencies are often ingrained and hard for fighters to change, making them more likely to appear in your fight as well.

Break Down Rounds: Pay attention to how your opponent's strategy evolves over the course of a fight. Some fighters start strong but lose steam, while others take a few rounds to find their rhythm. Breaking down each round can help you figure out when they're most vulnerable.

Assess Different Aspects Separately: Instead of trying to catch everything at once, focus on one area at a time. Watch a fight once to study footwork, another time to analyze hand positioning, and again to track defensive habits. This method allows you to pick up details you might miss if you're looking at everything at once.

Dissecting Defensive and Offensive Techniques

Understanding how your opponent defends and attacks is critical. Ask yourself:

Defensive Techniques: Do they rely more on slipping, blocking, or footwork to avoid punches? How do they react when cornered or pressured against the ropes? Do they drop their hands or make the same defensive move after throwing certain punches?

Offensive Combinations: What are their go-to combinations? Do they lead with a jab, then follow up with power punches? Do they repeatedly use the same counters? How do they set up their attacks, and can you identify any habits before they throw a punch?

Footwork and Movement

A fighter's footwork shows their strengths and weaknesses. Watch how they move around the ring—are they smooth and balanced, or do they cross their feet, giving you opportunities to attack? Look for moments when they're off-balance after throwing punches or when they change direction. Fighters who rely on speed or aggressive movement may put themselves in bad positions, especially when they're tired.

When watching their footwork, here's what to keep an eye on:

- Do they move in straight lines or pivot? Fighters who only move in straight lines are easier to trap and predict.

- Are they balanced after throwing combinations? If they lose their footing or stumble often, this is a good time to counter.

- Do they reset after attacking, or do they just keep charging forward? If they don't reset, they're vulnerable to quick counters, and may struggle with fighters who move well laterally.

- How well do they move side-to-side? Do they tend to favor one direction, constantly moving left or right? Recognizing a pattern in their movement allows you to anticipate their escape routes and cut them off more effectively.

Spotting these habits gives you chances to attack, counter, or control the pace of the fight.

Conditioning and Endurance

Some fighters start strong but get tired as the fight goes on. Studying your opponent's stamina is just as important as their skills. Do they slow down as the rounds progress, or do they start slow then pick up pace as the fight goes on? If you know when they tire, you can plan to push harder at the right time and take advantage when they're fatigued. If they start slow and gradually build momentum, you can exploit their early hesitation while ensuring you have the stamina to match their intensity when they shift gears.

Studying Your Own Footage

Just as you study your opponent, reviewing footage of yourself can be just as valuable. Watching your own fights and sparring sessions allows you to identify your own patterns, habits, and potential weaknesses. Are you overcommitting on certain punches and leaving yourself open? Are there predictable tendencies in your movement that an opponent could take advantage of? Studying yourself helps refine your skills and address areas that need improvement before your opponent can take advantage of them.

What if There's No Footage?

If you're an amateur, you won't always have footage of your opponent. In those cases, focus on your adaptability. Train to handle a variety of fighting styles so you're ready to adjust in the ring.

Here's how you can prepare:

Train to Face Different Styles:
Spar with fighters who have a range of fighting styles— aggressive punchers, defensive counter punchers, taller fighters, and those with longer reach. The more diverse your training partners, the better prepared you'll be to handle any situation in the ring.

Stay Flexible:

Without knowing your opponent's tendencies, you need to stay adaptable. In the first round, watch how they fight. Are they coming forward or staying back? Do they rely on certain punches or combinations? Adjust quickly and take advantage of what you see.

Trust Your Training:

The hard work you've put in during training will pay off. Go into the fight confident in your preparation, knowing that you've done everything you can to be ready.

Make Them React to You:

Even without footage, you can take control of the fight by making your opponent adjust to your style. Set the pace early, dictate the terms of the fight, and force them to react to your moves.

Lean on Your Team for Insights:

Your coach and team might have gathered valuable information about your opponent from other fighters or coaches. Listen closely to your corner during the fight, as they can spot things you might miss in the heat of the moment. Use the insights they provide to adjust your strategy as the fight progresses.

Chapter 14
Closing the Show: Becoming a Great Finisher

"I think I've become one of the best finishers in boxing; if I hurt a guy, I normally take him out." [25]
—Sugar Ray Leonard

The Difference Between a Predator and a Reckless Fighter

Finishing a fight means more than landing a big shot. It requires knowing when to press without leaving yourself open. A hurt opponent is still dangerous, sometimes even more so. They may throw wild counters, clinch desperately, or attempt to turn the momentum in their favor.

Many fighters make the mistake of rushing in the moment they see an opponent stumble, but reckless aggression can backfire. The best finishers don't rely on hope or emotion; they apply smart, systematic pressure, staying in control while methodically dismantling their opponent.

This chapter is about closing the show with calculated aggression and artistic violence. You'll learn how to break an opponent down, force mistakes, and execute the finish without burning yourself out or giving them a way back into the fight.

The Strategic Press: How to Apply Smart, Sustained Pressure

Strategic pressure isn't only for aggressive sluggers. It's a tool any fighter can use when the moment is right. Whether you're walking down a hurt opponent, pressing an elusive backfoot boxer, or looking to take control of the pace, smart pressure is about calculated control, not reckless aggression. Even fighters

---

[25] Sugar Ray Leonard made this comment in interview contexts, as collected in quote archives such as *BrainyQuote* and *AllGreatQuotes* (e.g., "I think I've become one of the best finishers in boxing...").

who typically move and counter can adopt this mindset when it's time to turn the tide.

Applying pressure is not about rushing in; it's about stalking with calculated intent. When cutting off the ring, don't follow, step into their exit routes and cut off their movement. Use half-steps instead of lunging forward, and maintain angles to keep them in range.

While pressing forward, you can throw with the intention of drawing out reactive counters from your opponent, and be fully prepared to counter their counter. This allows you to maintain pressure while staying defensively sharp and exploiting their desperation as they begin to break down.

Using tactical volume means throwing controlled combinations rather than wild flurries. Mixing up speed and power is what draws mistakes and makes you harder to defend against. Not every punch needs to be thrown at max effort.

Level changes play an important role in keeping an opponent guessing. A predictable headhunter is easy to defend against, while attacks that shift between high and low make defense much harder. Body shots are often overlooked, but consistent body work wears opponents down, making them less mobile and more vulnerable as the fight goes on.

The Setup Before the Finish

Finishes are rarely sudden. Most happen because an opponent has been systematically broken down, round by round. Fighters who understand this don't just chase a knockout; they gradually dissect their opponent until the stoppage becomes inevitable.

The key methods for breaking down an opponent include body work, measured dosages (controlled pacing of offense) and consistent mental/physical pressure. Targeting the body weakens their gas tank, slows movement, and forces their guard to drop, setting up clean shots to the head. Throwing too many punches too soon can drain your energy. Instead, pace your offense to stay effective throughout the fight. Steady pressure forces mistakes and limits your opponent's offense, not just by moving forward, but through feints, mental pressure, and a commanding presence that keeps them on edge.

When your opponent is in survival mode, cutting off the ring is a must. Instead of chasing, step into their exit routes to limit their movement, forcing them into positions where they have fewer options and must fight on your terms. Another key tactic is creating hesitation, making them second-guess their actions so they struggle to commit to their own offense. By recognizing their habits and disrupting their patterns, you can force predictable reactions and capitalize on them.

Baiting, probing, and feinting force reactions and create openings for clean shots. Staying defensively aware while maintaining offensive control ensures you're always ready to counter. Recognizing patterns in your opponent's movements and breaking them with speed changes and timing adjustments keeps you one step ahead.

How to Beat a Pressure Fighter by Flipping Their Strengths Against Them

To counteract a pressure fighter, pacing your offense is imperative. Don't get baited into throwing power shots repeatedly or throwing too many punches too early just to keep them off. Stay composed, pick shots wisely, and control the exchanges on your terms.

Body work is especially effective against a pressure fighter. They absorb punishment well, but attacking the body forces them to slow down and drains their stamina, ensuring they are not as fresh in the later rounds, where they typically thrive. Keeping them in check by making them respect your counters forces hesitation before they press forward, making them think twice before stepping into range.

Recognizing and disrupting a pressure fighter's habits and patterns is key. Instead of always reacting, use feints and traps to force them into mistakes. Angling and footwork, rather than simply backing up, allow you to pivot and sidestep, forcing the pressure fighter to reset rather than building momentum.

A pressure fighter wants their opponent to panic, exchange recklessly, or overwork themselves early. Instead, the key is to remain the calm, disciplined fighter who forces them to pay for every mistake. Slowing their work rate, making them hesitant, and controlling the fight on your terms is how pressure can be turned against them.

Once they are at the turning point, you can pick up the pace on them. The next section will explore the signs that the opponent will show when they are ready to be finished.

Signs an Opponent is Ready to Go

Recognizing the right moment to finish an opponent is just as important as knowing how to break them down. A fighter who is visibly hurt after taking a big shot—stumbling, freezing up, or reacting poorly—is often on the verge of being stopped. Slower reflexes, heavier breathing, and labored movements are clear signs that they are beginning to fade.

More clinching and backing up with no intent to counter indicate they are looking for a way out. Complaining to the ref or looking for a break in the action may also be a sign of exhaustion or discouragement. Spitting out the mouthpiece to buy time is another common tactic used to stall when hurt. Poor decision-making, throwing desperate shots or overcommitting, often signals that an opponent is breaking down mentally and physically.

A fading opponent will also be easier to hit continuously with minimal punches coming back. Not because they're backing off, but because they're being systematically broken down. At that point, they're more focused on weathering the storm than fighting back, leaving themselves open for sustained attacks.

Knowing when to press and when to ease off is something fighters develop through experience. It's about understanding their own gas tank and recognizing the right moments to capitalize on. The best finishers don't just attack blindly. They stay patient, picking the right time to close the show.

Not every fighter will be easy to finish, but this approach allows you to win rounds while steadily breaking them down. For amateurs with shorter fights or pros in the early stages of their career, this level of strategic energy management may not be as critical. However, as fights progress into 6-12 or 8-12 round bouts, the game shifts. Explosive power and speed alone won't carry a fighter through deep waters. Output must be controlled, pace dictated, and the opponent systematically worn down.

The Finisher's Mindset: Controlled Aggression vs. Recklessness

A wounded animal is still dangerous. A hurt fighter may throw wild counters in desperation or, in some cases, land a well-timed, drilled response, like Juan Manuel Marquez's perfectly placed counter against Manny Pacquiao in their fourth fight.

A desperate opponent might also clinch excessively to survive, forcing an overeager finisher to waste energy. Missing the opportunity to finish when the moment is right can give them a second wind, which can be dangerous. The key to finishing is balancing patience and urgency, pressing forward without overextending, keeping them reacting without lunging in blindly. Controlled aggression ensures excitement doesn't turn into reckless mistakes. Not every moment is worth chasing. A near-finish can be just as valuable if it wins you the round, breaks their confidence, or drains their gas tank.

Energy Management: Avoiding the "Redline"

Punching yourself out in a finishing attempt is one of the biggest dangers. Emptying the gas tank at the wrong time leaves you exposed, and if the finish isn't secured, it gives the opponent a new lifeline.

Instead of going full-throttle, attack in waves rather than one long burst. Controlled bursts allow for effective punches to land without overextending, then step back, reset, and re-enter.

Watch your opponent's body language closely. If the opponent isn't fighting back, the assault should continue. If they show signs of countering or weathering the storm, it's time to reset and adjust.

Mental exhaustion can be just as effective as physical fatigue. Opponents mentally break under constant, calculated pressure. When their confidence starts to crack, so does their ability to respond effectively. Mental fatigue leads to hesitation and stagnation, making them easier to break down physically.

As a fighter, you are the only one who truly knows where your redline is. You must learn to recognize when you're nearing that limit and make real-time decisions based on how your body feels in the moment. Whether you're closing in for a finish or maintaining an onslaught, only you can gauge how far to push, and when to pull back. The key is to finish smart, not rely on brute force alone.

Executing the Finish Without Getting Caught

Attacking from unexpected angles makes it harder for an opponent to survive. If they're shelling up, stepping to the side creates new openings for clean shots. Peels, pins, and posts (shown in chapter 12) can be used to manipulate their guard when they shell up, exposing targets that would otherwise be protected.

A desperate opponent will often resort to wild counters or clinching. If they start swinging recklessly, feinting to draw out their shot and countering is the safest response. If they clinch and one arm is freed, keep punching with that arm until they're forced to release the other. As soon as they let go, immediately switch hands and continue the attack, keeping them under fire, never giving them room to recover.

To break a stubborn grip in the clinch, a quick push–pull motion while stepping around the side can shift their balance and help loosen their hold. Framing (using your forearm or elbow to create space) on the inside or briefly tightening up before releasing can also create the space needed to strike or escape clean. Once you're free, circle to an angle and immediately reapply pressure, both mentally and physically.

If they're simply covering up, targeting the body with hooks and digging uppercuts through the middle will break their shell, forcing openings.

Round 3: The fighter's Mind

Chapter 15
The Psychology and Mental Game of Boxing

"There's one thing I don't ever think about: losing ...Instead, I think about how I'm going to win, and how I can do it the quickest way." [26]
—Joe Frazier

Boxing is more mental than people may realize. Joe Frazier didn't waste time thinking about losing, he obsessed over how to win. That mindset separated him from the pack. The body may throw the punches, but it's the mind that wins the fight.

Mindset: The Foundation of Champions

Your mindset either breaks you or builds you. It's the invisible weapon behind every comeback, every late-round surge, every moment a fighter refuses to fold. It shapes champions and drives fighters through their toughest battles. Muhammad Ali famously declared himself "The Greatest" before he had even earned the title, giving him a mental edge that pushed him to greatness. This level of self-belief is your greatest asset in the ring. A strong mindset can be as powerful as any physical skill in determining a fighter's success.

---

[26] Joe Frazier, interview and commentary, *Sports Illustrated*, March 15, 1971, in the feature article "The Battered Face of a Winner," published following his victory over Muhammad Ali at Madison Square Garden .

The Power of Self-Talk and "I Am" Affirmations

Feed your faith, starve your doubts

The voice inside your head can either propel you forward or hold you back. Imagine stepping into the ring with a mindset saying, "I'm the best," or "I am a beast" compared to "what am I doing here" or, "I hope I can do this." That voice in your head better be your ally, not your opponent. Talk like a killer, think like a winner. Your actions will follow.

Affirmations

Believing in your abilities primes you to perform at your absolute best. The way you talk to yourself can elevate your confidence and shape how you approach every challenge, especially when it becomes a daily habit.

Key Tips for Self-Talk

Be specific: Tailor your affirmations directly to your goals. For example, say, "I have the endurance to go all 10 rounds," to reinforce the mindset needed to perform at that level.

Use the present tense: Statements like "I'm a Beast" are far more powerful than saying "I will be determined". Affirm who you are in the present moment.

Visualize success: Pair your affirmations with mental imagery. Create a mental image of yourself executing your game plan flawlessly, from footwork to striking, reinforcing both your physical and mental preparation.

Handling Intimidation and Mental Warfare

Facing an intimidating opponent can stir fear, but maintaining a stoic mindset and focusing on your strengths helps you manage it. Opponents often use mind games to get inside your head. Trash talk can come from nerves or a desire to be entertaining, remember, they feel the same pressure you do. The key is to stay locked in on your strategy. Let your fists do the talking.

Thriving in Unfamiliar Sparring Settings

One of the best ways to strengthen your mental game is by sparring in unfamiliar settings. Stepping into a new gym, surrounded by strangers, and facing a sparring partner you know nothing about can bring on those familiar "butterfly" feelings. The uncertainty of what to expect can trigger anxiety or self-doubt, but these feelings are a natural part of growth. It's in these moments that the mental game is won.

In my own career, I made it a point to travel and spar in gyms where I was the outsider, facing new opponents who I knew little about. Those sessions always brought a rush of nerves, but they taught me more than any controlled environment ever could. *(They were also great for networking and building connections—most of my biggest opportunities came through relationships I built while sparring in those gyms.)*

There is also the pressure to perform. Being the visitor, the competitive nature kicks in fast. You want to earn respect. You want to show you belong. That pressure sharpens you, and it teaches you how to perform when it counts.

Just like walking into the ring, walking into an unknown gym requires you to face the fear of the unknown head-on. The uncertainty of not knowing how your opponent will move or how they'll react to your attacks mirrors the unpredictability of fight night. By testing myself in these environments, I built the confidence and mental toughness necessary to think under pressure and develop comfort in the ring.

This kind of sparring is about learning how to perform when the situation isn't ideal and when nerves are running high. The more you expose yourself to these situations, the more you train your mind to stay calm, focus on the task, and overcome the discomfort. It's just another form of preparation, one that doesn't always happen in the comfort of your own gym, but rather in the real world, where you'll have to thrive regardless of the circumstances.

Staying Calm Under Pressure

The mark of a true champion is the ability to stay calm in the storm. Whether it's in a heated exchange or in the moments before the fight, controlling your emotions gives you the ability to focus on the task at hand.

> *"I'm never angry in the ring, never stressed. And that's important, because that emotional control helps me to pay attention to the details. If you're stressed, you can't do that. But I can."* [27]
> —Mikey Garcia, a four-weight world champion

Techniques to Restore Calm in the Ring:

Reset with Controlled Breathing: If you feel yourself tensing up, take a deep breath in through your nose, then exhale slowly. A controlled exhale relaxes your nervous system, keeping you sharp instead of panicked. Do this between rounds or in brief lulls during the fight.

Micro-Pauses for Composure: If the fight starts to feel overwhelming, take a brief moment to reset. Step back, circle away, or clinch for a second to regain control of your breathing and refocus.

---

[27] Garcia, Mikey. Quote from pre-fight interview discussing his approach to emotional control in boxing. Garcia is a former four-division world champion known for his technical precision and ring IQ, though no exact source for this specific phrasing could be located.

Tension Check: Fighters often burn unnecessary energy by staying too tense. Do a quick mental scan of your body. Relax your shoulders, unclench your fists, and stay loose. The more relaxed you are, the sharper and faster your reactions will be.

Command Your Self-Talk: Instead of letting frustration or fear creep in, reinforce calm with short, direct cues like, "Stay sharp," "I control the pace," or, "I see everything." Your internal voice is as important as any physical adjustment.

Practicing Composure in Training:

Spar with a Purpose: Set rounds where the goal is to remain calm under pressure. For example, spar an aggressive partner but focus on controlled breathing and staying relaxed under fire.

Train Fatigued: Practice executing technique and decision-making when exhausted so fight-night pressure doesn't feel unfamiliar. Push yourself in training, then force yourself to breathe, reset, and execute.

Embrace the Chaos: Instead of trying to eliminate nerves, accept them and turn them into focus. Remind yourself: "I trained for this. I thrive under pressure."

The Confidence of a Winner

It all begins in the mind. If you don't believe in your abilities, how can you perform at your best? Your body follows your mind, and it performs around the beliefs you carry deep within. It's normal to feel doubts. Outwork them. Let your preparation bury your uncertainty. Here's the truth: When you physically FEEL like a beast, that inner self-confidence comes naturally, because the only way to reach that level is through relentless effort and discipline.

Confidence isn't something you fake or force. It's built through work. Real work. Not talking about it. Not pretending. Just showing up, grinding, and doing it when nobody else is.

When you step in the ring and *know* you did everything, that confidence becomes unshakable.

Confidence comes from competence. The more skilled and prepared you are, the more naturally confident you become. When you've trained hard and have left no stones unturned, hesitation fades, and execution takes over.

Flip the script. Instead of worrying about what your opponent is going to do, or what might happen if you lose, shift the focus. They have to worry about you. They have to deal with everything you're bringing into this fight. Remind yourself: "I already won this in the gym."

It's important to respect your opponent as a threat, but never forget, your hard work will speak for itself.

Be careful what you say. Words carry power. Be conscious of the language you speak into existence. It makes more of a difference than most realize.

Believing in Yourself When Others Don't

> *"To be a champion, you must believe in yourself when nobody else will."* [28] —Sugar Ray Robinson

What I'm saying is to have extreme self-belief. Some pessimists may call it 'delusional'. But simply put, it's not delusional if you put the work in.

There will be times when others doubt you, but remember, this is your journey. Keep believing in yourself, even when no one else does. The ability to push forward, even when faced with doubt, is what will set you apart from the rest.

---

[28] Sugar Ray Robinson, quoted in *Sports Illustrated*, "A Punch for History," May 13, 1957.

To train an unshakable mind, you must build mental habits. Use gratitude to counter negativity, discipline to override laziness, and detachment to reduce mental distress. Just as the body grows stronger through repeated resistance, the mind becomes more resilient through daily training. And that's where discipline takes over.

The Power of Discipline

"To be the best, you have to put in overtime." [29] —Floyd Mayweather Jr.

Once the mind is forged, it's time to align it with disciplined action. Mindset alone won't carry you... your habits must back it up. That's where the power of discipline comes in.

Discipline is the silent force behind success in boxing. Legends like Muhammad Ali and Julio Cesar Chavez knew that hard work and consistency would shape them into champions. Chavez Sr. famously said, "The key to success in boxing is discipline and perseverance." Ali added to this idea, stating, "Suffer now and live the rest of your life as a champion." This unwavering dedication drove them to outwork their competition and stay committed to their craft.

Mike Tyson put it bluntly: "Discipline is doing what you hate to do, but doing it like you love it." Even the toughest fighters have to push through tasks they don't enjoy, but it's their mindset and dedication that set them apart.

Discipline means consistently showing up. Whether it's late night runs, strict diets, or relentless training. It's about pushing through when you're tired and staying focused despite distractions. Without discipline, even the most talented fighters fall short.

This all sounds great, but how do I get motivated or force myself to be disciplined? Well, discipline doesn't rely on motivation, it

---

[29] Mayweather Jr., Floyd. Quote from "All Access: Mayweather vs. Canelo" documentary series, Showtime Sports, Episode 1, 2013. This reflected his well-known "hard work, dedication" philosophy.

comes from having a system. Set up your day so that certain actions happen automatically: wake up, hydrate, get your run in, eat clean, and stick to your training schedule.

Use discipline triggers. These are simple cues that kick off your routine without needing to think. That could be laying out your wraps and gloves the night before, stepping on the scale first thing in the morning, logging your session and looking at your training journal, or even setting a motivational ringtone for your alarm so that's the first thing that enters your mind. These cues tell your brain, it's time to lock in.

And anytime you're torn between a choice, whether it's skipping your run, eating something you know isn't helping you, or hitting snooze instead of getting after it—ask yourself: "Will my future self be proud of this decision?"

That simple question can cut through the noise. Discipline is just stacking decisions your future self will thank you for.

With that said, discipline doesn't need to feel like a daily battle. You don't overthink it, you just go. Action creates momentum. And that momentum starts the cycle.

The goal is to build a rhythm. When you take action, you get a small win. That win creates motivation. That motivation leads to more action. The cycle feeds itself, and over time, it becomes who you are. When you start to see the results of just showing up and putting in this work, that progress creates a powerful drive to keep going. It stops being a grind and starts becoming something you look forward to.

With repetition, discipline turns into habit. And once it's a habit... It's automatic.

Crafting a Champion's Routine

"It's tough to get out of bed to do roadwork at 5AM when you've been sleeping in silk pajamas." [30]—Marvin Hagler

Building discipline starts with a routine. Grueling boxing workouts, cardio, strength training, and a balanced diet are the foundation of a fighter's day. A structured routine eliminates distractions and keeps you focused.

Laser Focus: The Key to Greatness

Discipline builds the base. Focus sharpens the blade. The fighters who go far are the ones who stay locked in while everyone else is drifting. True champions live and breathe boxing, sacrificing everything else for their pursuit of greatness.

Eliminating Distractions: To succeed, you must remove anything that doesn't contribute to your success. This might mean sacrificing relationships, hobbies, or other interests to stay focused on your goals.

With discipline and focus in place, the next level is mental clarity. And in boxing, a clear mind is just as dangerous as a sharp jab.

Zen in the Ring: Meditation

Chaos is part of the fight. The ones who last know how to stay calm in it. When the pressure's on, clarity wins. Meditation builds that clarity. It trains your mind to stay sharp, steady and in control, no matter what's coming at you.

---

[30] Hagler, Marvin. Interview with Ring Magazine, 1987. Discussing the challenges of maintaining hunger and drive after achieving success.

The Practice of Meditation: A Fighter's Guide

Find a Quiet Space: Sit comfortably in a peaceful environment where you won't be interrupted.

Anchor with Breath: Inhale deeply, exhale slowly. Let the breath center you, like a steady rhythm in the chaos of a fight.

Clear Your Mind: When your thoughts wander, gently bring your focus back to your breath. This mirrors the way you refocus between rounds.

Start Small: Begin with just a few minutes a day, and gradually increase the duration as it becomes a part of your routine.

End with Intention: Set a powerful affirmation to guide your day. Say, *"I am focused and will stay locked in while training today."* Use it as a focus point throughout your sessions.

The Benefits: Mental Strength for the Ring

Enhanced Focus: Teaches your mind to stay in the present, sharpening your reactions and timing in the ring.

Stress Reduction: Lowers anxiety, enabling you to perform with a clear mind under pressure.

Mental Toughness: Builds the endurance to push through tough moments in training and fights.

Emotional Control: Helps you stay composed, preventing emotions from disrupting your strategy.

Visualization: The Mental Edge

Visualization is how you rehearse the chaos before it happens. So when the moment comes, your body already knows what to do.

Muhammad Ali used it like a weapon. He *saw* the outcome before the first punch was thrown. Victory wasn't a surprise. It was a replay.

Ali sometimes predicted the exact round he would win, envisioning every punch, every slip, every moment before it happened. His bold predictions weren't just for show, they were the result of hours spent seeing it all unfold in his mind. By the time he stepped into the ring, the outcome already felt familiar.

Conor McGregor, also known during this time as "The Mystic Mac," took a similar approach. He visualized every detail. His walk to the cage, the first exchange, the shot that would end it. There were times it played out exactly how he saw it. That kind of belief doesn't come from hype. It comes from seeing it so many times in your head that your body starts to follow the script.

Sugar Ray Leonard was another master of visualization. Before every fight, he'd run the whole thing in his mind. Combinations, slips, the flow of the fight, how he'd stay composed under fire. He didn't leave anything to chance. So when it was time to perform, his reactions were sharp, automatic, and instinctive. That edge made the difference.

The Science Behind Visualization

Visualization is beyond mental imagery, it rewires the brain. A study by Dr. Blaslotto at the University of Chicago divided participants into three groups:

- One group practiced shooting free throws physically.
- Another group visualized making successful free throws.
- The third group did nothing.

After 30 days, the group that practiced physically improved by 24%. Remarkably, the group that only visualized improved by 23%, nearly matching the physically practicing group (Blaslotto et al., 1996). This study demonstrates that visualization can nearly replicate the physical effects of practice, showing just how powerfully the brain can rehearse and refine movement—even without physical action.

Why Visualization Works

Strengthens Neural Connections: Reinforces muscle memory, making movements smoother and more instinctive.

Builds Confidence: Mentally rehearsing success eliminates doubt and primes you for peak performance.

Manages Pressure: Visualizing scenarios prepares you to stay calm, no matter what unfolds in the ring.

How to Visualize: Engage All Your Senses

Effective visualization is more than imagining success, it's about immersing yourself fully in the experience. Engage every sense to make the mental rehearsal as vivid as possible.

1. **See** yourself moving with precision and landing clean punches.

2. **Feel** the tension in your muscles, the snap of each punch, and the sweat on your skin.

3. **Hear** the crowd's roar, your coach's instructions, and the sound of gloves landing.

4. **Smell** the familiar scent of leather, sweat, and the gym environment.

5. **Taste** the sweetness of victory as you visualize your hand being raised.

Don't just see the fight. Make it real in your mind, so your body already knows what to do when it happens. Ali, McGregor, and Leonard mentally rehearsed their success until it felt inevitable. By the time they entered the ring or octagon, they had already won the fight in their minds.

Winning on Repeat: The Power of Consistent Visualization

Visualization is not a one-time practice. It's a habit that builds over time. Each session strengthens the connection between your mind and body, making your movements feel natural and instinctive when it matters most.

Ali's predictions weren't by coincidence, he had already fought and won in his mind. McGregor's flawless performances reflected the power of this. Leonard's ability to remain calm under pressure came from visualizing even the toughest moments. These athletes understood that success begins in the mind.

When you visualize success repeatedly and with detail, your mind begins to accept that outcome as normal. Your body follows suit, executing with precision and confidence, because it's already been there countless times.

Commit to daily visualization. Step into the ring knowing you've already been there. Mentally, emotionally, physically.

Meditation and Visualization: A Powerful Duo

When combined, meditation and visualization elevate your mental preparation to new heights. Meditation clears your mind, making it more open and receptive to visualization. In this calm, focused state, you can vividly picture yourself executing techniques, staying composed under pressure, and achieving success in the ring.

With consistent practice, this process taps into your subconscious mind, creating automatic habits that become second nature. Mental rehearsals reinforce your instincts, so your actions flow seamlessly under pressure. Over time, these repetitions sharpen your reactions, allowing you to perform without hesitation. Focused, precise, and fully in control.

Fight Day Mindset: Trusting Your Training and Enjoying the Moment

"It's just a job. Grass grows, birds fly, waves pound the sand. I beat people up."
[31]—Muhammad Ali

By the time fight day arrives, you've done the hard work. You've trained, prepared, and honed your skills. Trust in your training, and let your body perform as it's been conditioned to. Your movements should be automatic, a result of countless hours of practice.

Tips for Fight Day

Unconscious Competence: Trust that your body knows what to do. Let instincts take over and reactions fire without hesitation.

Have Fun: The hard work is done. Now it's time to enjoy the thrill of the fight. Feel the crowd. Breathe it in. Lock eyes with your opponent like you've already seen the ending. You trained for this. Now deliver.

Stay Calm and Focused: Use controlled breathing and stay locked into the present moment. Let your mind stay clear and sharp. Remember, your opponent is feeling the same emotions and nerves. They're human, too. Confidence isn't about having no nerves, it's about managing them better than your opponent.

---

[31] Ali, Muhammad. Pre-fight interview before his bout with George Foreman, "The Rumble in the Jungle," Kinshasa, Zaire (now Democratic Republic of the Congo), October 1974.

Positive Self-Talk: Remind yourself of your strengths with affirmations like, *"I'm relentless,"* or, *"Nobody works as hard as me."* Instead of saying, *"I'm nervous,"* try saying, *"I'm excited, and this adrenaline is here to help me focus."*

When your preparation, discipline, and mindset are in sync, execution isn't something you have to think about. It just happens.

Final Thoughts

Boxing is as much a mental game as it is a physical one. The foundation of success starts with disciplined preparation: Relentless training, strategic planning, and physical conditioning. But a fighter's greatest weapon isn't just their body, it's their mind.

The fighters who last are the ones with a mind of steel. When you train your mind through meditation, visual reps, and ruthless self-talk, you become dangerous before the bell even rings. Stack that with real discipline and preparation... you're a problem nobody wants to solve.

Once you've built the foundation of mental resilience, focus, and confidence, something else kicks in. You stop thinking, you just flow. That's when greatness shows up. Not forced. Automatic.

Enter: Flow State.

Chapter 16
Enter The Matrix: Unlocking Flow State

"The best moments in our lives are not the passive, receptive, relaxing times... The best moments usually occur if a person's body or mind is stretched to its limits in a voluntary effort to accomplish something difficult and worthwhile." [32]
—Mihaly Csikszentmihalyi

Have you ever been so absorbed in an activity that time seemed to slip away and everything else faded into the background? This deep focus and heightened awareness is what experts call the flow state. Imagine yourself in the ring, effortlessly dodging punches and landing combinations with perfect precision, as if time itself has slowed down. It's like being in the Matrix, where every movement feels instinctive and perfectly timed. Achieving this state can elevate your performance to its highest level, whether in training or competition.

The concept of 'flow' was introduced by psychologist Mihaly Csikszentmihalyi in the 1970s. He studied how artists, musicians, and athletes described being fully immersed and energized by their work, which led to peak performance.

Minimizing Distractions

To reach a flow state, it's important to eliminate distractions, both external and internal. That could mean the noise from the crowd, overthinking your last sparring session, or that voice in your head trying to pull your focus somewhere else. Setting clear goals for each training session or fight helps focus your mind. Techniques like deep breathing, mindfulness, and visualization

---

[32] Mihaly Csikszentmihalyi, *Flow: The Psychology of Optimal Experience* (New York: Harper & Row, 1990), 3–4.

can bring you back to the present moment, allowing you to stay sharp and fully engaged.

Balancing Challenge and Skill

Flow occurs when you're faced with just the right level of challenge, where your skills are pushed but not overwhelmed. In boxing, this balance can come from sparring with different opponents, learning advanced techniques, or pushing through intense training. You don't grow when it's easy. And you don't flow when you're drowning. Flow state lives in between the two.

Preparation, Recovery, and Flow: The Formula for Peak Performance

Train with purpose. Recover with intention. Fight on instinct. That's how you enter flow. With a rested body and clear mind, you can instinctively read your opponent and react without much thought. It's this balance of preparation, recovery, and sharp focus that unlocks the flow state, allowing you to perform at your absolute peak when it matters most.

Flow sharpens your focus, improves reaction time, and heightens your ability to perform under pressure. For a boxer, being in this state means landing punches with accuracy, anticipating your opponent's moves, and staying composed throughout the fight. Your mind slows down while your body speeds up. Flow helps you make smarter decisions, stay calm under fire, and operate at the highest level in the ring.

When you're in flow, every movement feels natural, and time seems to slow down. Athletes across all disciplines seek this state because it leads to peak performance. Preparation builds it. Recovery unlocks it. Focus allows it to take over. By focusing on preparation and recovery, you'll position yourself to enter flow on fight night, allowing you to perform at your best when it counts.

Chapter 17
The Alter Ego: Forged in Training Camp

Who you are in the ring isn't always who you are outside of it. That version of you is built for war. And it's forged in fire. In the world of combat sports, physical training, skill, and strategy are often emphasized as the keys to success. But beneath the surface lies another powerful tool, one that can take your performance to a completely different level: your alter ego. This chapter explores how this identity change is created, shaped and strengthened during the intense process of training and fight camp preparation.

The Power of the Alter Ego

An alter ego—a psychological concept of an alternative self—isn't simply a flashy nickname or a persona used for intimidation; it's a mental shift that allows fighters to tap into traits and abilities that may not always surface in everyday life. It becomes a source of focus, aggression, and resilience that can push you beyond your limits. Training camp provides the perfect environment for this transformation, as both your body and mind are tested like never before.

An alter ego gives you the ability to separate who you are outside the ring from who you become inside it. This mental separation allows fighters to shed any doubts, fears, or hesitations, and adopt a mindset that is relentless, fearless, and focused solely on victory.

You don't have to actively create an alter ego, but through concentrated and consistent training, a different part of you is being formed, a more focused and resilient version of yourself. This transformation happens naturally, as it should, and must, through the intense challenges you face in preparation. You tap into and feed this part of yourself during training, sparring, and competition, allowing it to grow stronger each time.

For some fighters, consciously creating an alter ego can be a powerful option when the feelings of fear, anxiety, or pressure become overwhelming. It's not mandatory, but deliberately stepping into a crafted persona can help channel those emotions into controlled aggression and focus, turning nervous energy into fuel.

Let's look at how some of the greatest fighters in history have harnessed this tool to become legends in the sport.

Real Fighters, Real Alter Egos

Muhammad Ali–"The Greatest": Ali didn't just believe he was the best, he told the world. "The Greatest" wasn't just a nickname; it was an alter ego that allowed Ali to step into the ring with supreme confidence, no matter who he was facing. This mental shift gave him an edge, helping him rise to any occasion, block out fear, and perform with the swagger of a champion, even in the most challenging moments. Ali's alter ego allowed him to stay sharp and keep his focus on the fight, not the distractions.

Mike Tyson–"Iron Mike": When Tyson walked into the ring as "Iron Mike", he transformed into a force of raw, destructive power. His alter ego reflected pure aggression, and it helped him intimidate opponents long before the fight even started. "Iron Mike" represented the primal, unstoppable side of Tyson's fighting style, a persona that allowed him to channel his rage and strength into calculated, devastating punches. Tyson's persona turned him into someone whose presence broke opponents before the first punch. Tyson himself has said, "The closer I get to the ring the more confident I get. Once I'm in the ring, I'm a God." This transformation symbolized his complete mental and physical dominance, turning him into a cold, explosive weapon with one mission... destruction.

Deontay Wilder–"The Bronze Bomber": Wilder's alter ego, "The Bronze Bomber", was a deliberate creation, a persona meant to symbolize his relentless pursuit of knockouts. The Bronze Bomber wasn't just about winning; it was about leaving his opponents completely unconscious on the canvas. Wilder's alter ego allowed him to tap into his most aggressive instincts while maintaining focus on his ultimate goal: destruction in the ring. This separation of his personal life from his fighting life gave him the mental space to focus purely on victory, knowing that in the ring, he was a different person. A cold-blooded knockout artist.

"Sugar" Ray Leonard: Leonard famously explained the power of his alter ego: "When I looked in the mirror before the fight, if I saw 'Sugar' Ray Leonard in the mirror, I was invincible. If I saw Ray Leonard, it was going to be a tough night." This clear distinction between his personal self and his alter ego gave him an edge in the ring. As "Sugar" Ray Leonard, he became a sharper, more locked-in version of himself. A fighter who stayed calm, calculated, and always found a way to win. This warrior spirit allowed him to enter the ring with complete confidence and control, knowing that when he became "Sugar" he was at his best.

Tyson Fury–"The Gypsy King": Fury's "Gypsy King" alter ego reflects his heritage and warrior spirit. This persona has helped him overcome personal struggles and dominate in the ring. Fury said, "Alter egos are often bigger versions of yourself. If you were to walk out onto a stage in front of tens of thousands of people, to capture everyone's attention, you will need to be commanding or free from fear and stage fright. By becoming a supreme version of yourself, who moves and talks in a different way, you can overcome your own self-doubting personality and take on a more confident character." This mental approach has allowed Fury to thrive under the spotlight and overcome immense challenges both inside and outside the ring.

Marvin Hagler–"Marvelous": He was so frustrated that commentators refused to call him by his nickname that he legally changed his name to "Marvelous Marvin Hagler." Hagler became the "Marvelous" persona, often referring to the "monster" inside him that would take over in the ring. This alter ego channeled his aggression and focus, making him a relentless champion who could destroy his opponents with unwavering determination.

Kobe Bryant–"Black Mamba": Though a basketball player, Bryant's "Black Mamba" alter ego is a powerful example of how adopting a fierce and focused persona can drive an athlete to excellence. "Black Mamba" was Bryant's way of becoming hyper-focused, deadly, and resilient. Someone who could execute under immense pressure.

The Brutal Realities of the Sport

> *"Boxing is the only sport you can get your brain shook, your money took and your name in the undertaker's book."* [33]
> –Joe Frazier

Boxing is one of the most demanding and brutal sports, requiring not only physical strength but also immense mental resilience. The realities of stepping into the ring, facing pain, potential injury, and the psychological warfare of competition, can be overwhelming. An alter ego can serve as a vital coping mechanism, helping fighters to mentally armor themselves against the harsh realities of the sport. It allows them to step into a role where fear and hesitation are replaced by determination and aggression.

Training Camp as the Forge of the Alter Ego

Training camp is where the fighter inside you is hardened through exhaustion, repetition, and relentless mental pressure. The structure and discipline of camp strips away distractions, forcing you to tap into the version of yourself that refuses to break, quit, or hesitate.

---

[33] Joe Frazier, quoted in *The Soul of a Butterfly: Reflections on Life's Journey* by Muhammad Ali and Hana Yasmeen Ali (New York: Simon & Schuster, 2004), 103.

This is where the alter ego is truly formed. Not in the moment of victory, but in the unseen, grueling hours of training with no applause.

Isolation and Focus: Training camp forces fighters into a singular focus, shutting out the outside world so that the fighter's persona can take full control.

Pushing Beyond Limits: Fatigue, pain, and mental battles forge the alter ego's resilience, so that when the moment of truth comes, you have supreme confidence.

Embracing the Role: Repetition ingrains new instincts, sharper reflexes, and a relentless mindset, reinforcing the fighter's identity separate from their everyday self.

This transformation can generally happen in training camp, where exhaustion forces you to dig deeper than you thought possible. Every round, every grueling session, you are feeding that persona, shaping it, becoming it. The specifics of structuring a training camp are covered in Chapter 21 (*Training Camp: The Blueprint for Fight Readiness*), but here, the focus is on the psychological shift. How camp forges the mindset that carries you into battle.

Step Into Your Supreme Self

Fury's insight about the "supreme version of yourself" demonstrates that adopting an alter ego is not about pretending to be someone you're not, it's about stepping into the most confident, commanding version of yourself. The key lies in creating a mental shift that allows you to shed hesitation and fear, replacing them with focus, aggression, and resilience. Whether you're preparing for a fight or simply looking to elevate your performance, this process can transform how you approach both training and competition. Let's break down how you can build and strengthen your own alter ego, step by step.

Creating Your Alter Ego: A Practical Guide

Define the Traits of Your Alter Ego

Take a moment to think about the qualities you need most in the ring. Is it fearlessness? Unwavering focus? Aggression? This persona should have the traits that push you beyond your limits and help you thrive under pressure.

Prompt: Write down three traits that describe the fighter you want to become. Look at it before you train. Let it remind you what kind of fighter you're building.

Give Your Alter Ego a Name

Names are powerful. By naming this identity, you give it life and separate it from your everyday self. This name could be a reflection of your fighting style, mindset, or a characteristic you aspire to embody.

Example: Just as Muhammad Ali became "The Greatest" and Tyson Fury embraced "The Gypsy King", you can craft a persona that reflects your unique strengths.

Prompt: Spend a few minutes brainstorming names that resonate with your fighting identity. Choose one that feels empowering and personal.

Establish Rituals to Trigger Your Alter Ego

Rituals act as mental switches that help you step into this mindset. These could be as simple as wrapping your hands, listening to a specific song, or even visualizing yourself as your alter ego before training or sparring.

Practical Example: Before stepping into the gym, play a specific playlist that pumps you up and signals the mental shift.

Prompt: Identify one or two rituals you can perform consistently to activate your alter ego.

Visualize Your Alter Ego in Action

Visualization is one of the most powerful tools for stepping into this mental shift. Before training, take a few minutes to close your eyes and picture yourself as your alter ego —how you move, how you react under pressure, and how you dominate in the ring.

Practical Exercise

At the start of every session, spend two to three minutes imagining this version of yourself walking into the gym, owning the space, and executing with precision.

1. **Affirmations**: Reinforce this visualization with affirmations like, "I have heightened awareness in the ring," or, "My defense is impeccable, and my punches are sharp and accurate."

2. **Sparring as Your Alter Ego:** Sparring is the ideal environment to bring this mindset to life. Use these sessions to fully tap into the aggression, calmness, or focus it represents. Pay attention to how this mental shift impacts your performance.

Tip: If your alter ego is about remaining calm under pressure, consciously focus on staying composed even when you're fatigued or under heavy attack.

3. **Reflect and Refine:** Your alter ego isn't static. It evolves with you. After each training session or sparring match, reflect on how well you mentally locked in and what you can adjust.

Prompt: Ask yourself, "Did I bring my alter ego into the session? How can I channel it more effectively next time?"

What If You're an Amateur or Have Limited Time?

While a full, immersive training camp is the ideal environment for developing an alter ego, fighters with limited time or balancing other responsibilities can still apply the core principles. By focusing on condensed, high-intensity sessions and incorporating visualization and mental training into their daily lives, they can still unlock their alter ego when it matters most. The tips for creating your alter ego, above, can still apply.

The key is to maximize focus during whatever time you do have, both in the gym and mentally. Even short bursts of intense preparation can help you build that mindset and let it take over when it's time to fight.

Carve out small moments throughout your day to strengthen this mindset. Spend 10 minutes in the morning visualizing yourself as your alter ego, use your commute or downtime to reinforce this shift, whether by listening to a playlist that gets you in the right headspace, repeating key affirmations, or mentally walking through fight scenarios, and rehearse your alter ego's mindset while wrapping your hands before training. These small but intentional habits reinforce the transformation, making it second nature when it's time to perform.

Flip the Switch

Creating and channeling an alter ego can be a game-changer in your journey to becoming a world-class fighter. It allows you to tap into hidden reserves of strength, focus, and confidence, providing the mental edge necessary for success. Remember, this transformation is not about pretending to be someone else but about unlocking the most powerful version of yourself when it matters most. Interweave it into your psyche, and let it guide you to greatness once the bell rings. When the lights are on, you don't need to think. You just become.

Chapter 18
Transforming Fear into Courage

"The hero and the coward both feel the same thing. But the hero uses his fear, projects it onto his opponent, while the coward runs. It's the same thing, fear, but it's what you do with it that matters." [34]—Cus D'Amato

In boxing, just like in life, fear is always present. Fear of being hit. Fear of failure. Fear of injury. Even the fear of letting people down. This chapter will dive into how fear can impact you and how to turn it into something that helps you instead of holding you back.

Understanding Fear

Fear is natural and necessary. It kept our ancestors alive. But in boxing, it can stop you from reaching your full potential. It can cloud your judgment, make decisions harder, and slow you down in the ring. To beat fear, you need to understand it and control it.

Fear can hurt you by:

- Clouding your judgment.
- Making decisions harder.
- Hurting your performance.

But fear can also be your fuel. When controlled, it helps you:

- Focus more.
- Work harder.
- Stay disciplined.

Identifying Fear Triggers

Every boxer feels fear differently. It's important to figure out what exactly triggers yours. Is it a skilled opponent? A large

---

[34] D'Amato, Cus, quoted in *Iron Ambition: My Life with Cus D'Amato* by Mike Tyson and Larry Sloman (New York: Blue Rider Press, 2017), 54.

audience? Identifying the things that make you afraid is the first step to overcoming them.

Pre-Fight Jitters

> *"Everyone gets butterflies before a big game. Champions get 'em all going in the same direction and use them for energy, not anxiety."* [35]— Tim Grover

Even the best fighters get nervous before a match. It's completely normal. The hours leading up to a fight can fill you with anxiety. But nerves don't have to control you. Use techniques like deep breathing, visualization, or meditation. These will calm your mind and body, shifting your focus from fear to the fight ahead.

Using Fear as Fuel

The legendary coach Cus D'Amato said: "Boxing is a sport of self-control. You must understand fear so you can manipulate it. Fear is like fire. You can make it work for you."

Fear can be a powerful motivator. It can push you to train harder, focus more, and stay disciplined. Mike Tyson, often called "The Baddest Man on the Planet", used fear to fuel his training. He admitted that fear kept him disciplined, making him work harder and stay sharp. If someone as fierce as Tyson felt fear, it shows that fear is normal. But by using it to fuel his preparation, Tyson increased his chances of winning.

Fear of losing or getting hurt can drive you to perform better. Channel that fear into your preparation, and it can elevate your game. It makes you mentally tougher and physically stronger.

Harnessing the Power of Fear

Fear isn't weakness, it's raw fuel. It's energy waiting for direction. Understanding your fear allows you to turn it into

---

[35] Grover, Tim. *Relentless: From Good to Great to Unstoppable*. Scribner, 2013.

something positive: focus, discipline, and work ethic. Overcoming fear takes time, but once you master it, you unlock new potential, both in and out of the ring.

Techniques for Channeling Fear into Power:

Fight-Day Breathing: Take slow, controlled breaths (inhale for four seconds, hold for four, exhale for four, repeat) to slow your heart rate and reduce nerves. As previously mentioned, deep breathing stabilizes your nervous system, keeping you focused and composed.

Visualization Rehearsal: Close your eyes and mentally walk through your fight. Imagine yourself executing sharp movements, controlling the ring, and responding to pressure with confidence. The brain struggles to distinguish between real and imagined experiences, so rehearsing success reduces fear's grip.

The "Present Moment" Reset: Fear thrives on "what if" thinking. What if I get hit? What if I lose? Combat this by anchoring yourself in the present moment. Feel your fists clench, notice the floor beneath your feet, and focus on your breathing. This keeps fear from gaining control.

Pre-Fight Mantras: Many elite fighters use self-talk to reframe fear. Instead of, "I'm nervous," say, "I'm ready. My training is my weapon." A simple but powerful phrase can shift your mindset from fear to confidence.

Action Over Anxiety: Fear weakens when you move. Shadowbox, skip rope, or throw light punches before a fight to channel nervous energy into action and warm up your muscles. Once you start moving, hesitation fades.

Chapter 19
Injuries and Losses: Turning Setbacks into Strength

"Tough times don't last, tough people do." [36]
—Robert H. Schuller, motivational speaker

Injuries and losses are challenges that athletes of all sports encounter on their journey. They can knock you down, mess with your confidence, and make you question everything. But here's the thing: setbacks, while painful, are where real growth happens. If you handle them right, they can make you stronger, sharper, and more resilient than ever. As Ryan Holiday says, *The obstacle is the way.*[37] These setbacks aren't roadblocks, they are the path to your progress.

Dealing with Injuries

The first step to overcoming any injury? Face it head-on. Don't try to push through the pain or ignore it. Accept that you're hurt, and seek medical attention right away. A solid diagnosis and a plan for recovery are your new playbook. Stick to it religiously, because rushing back too soon can mess you up even worse in the long run.

Just like consistency drives improvement in training, consistency in your recovery is what ensures you come back stronger. You must approach recovery with the same discipline that you bring to training. Healing is just another part of the process. One that demands patience.

I learned this firsthand when I suffered a blunt force injury to my leg while sparring a heavyweight. It was an accidental shot,

---

[36] Schuller, Robert H. From "Tough Times Never Last, but Tough People Do!" (1983). The phrase has since become a widely used motivational maxim in sports and beyond.

[37] Aurelius, Marcus. "Meditations," Book 5, Section 20, circa 170-180 CE. Roman Emperor and Stoic philosopher. Quote popularized in modern times by Ryan Holiday's book "The Obstacle Is the Way" (2014).

but in hindsight, it was foolish on my part to be sparring a heavyweight to begin with. At first, it felt like just a minor ache, something I could train through. But over time, the pain worsened, leading to severe issues bending my leg.

I ignored it and kept training for a fight against Olympic bronze medalist and former world champion Yordenis Ugas, a proud Cuban technician known for his skill and sharp counterpunching ability.

I continued training through swimming and shadowboxing, doing my best to avoid putting too much stress on my leg. I didn't want to back out. I had already been forced to reschedule that fight once due to a fractured thumb. I took my first professional loss in that fight, and afterward, I finally got an X-ray and found out I had developed myositis ossificans, a condition where bone starts forming inside muscle due to blunt trauma. That was a lesson in itself: listen to your body. Pushing through can sometimes cost more in the long run.

Staying Active and Adapting

Being sidelined doesn't mean you're out of the game. Even with an injury, there are ways to stay active within safe limits. Hurt your hand? Work the other hand. Injured your arm? Focus on lower-body strength and conditioning. Low-impact activities like yoga or meditation can help maintain balance and mental sharpness.

I didn't rest, I adapted. During my recovery from myositis ossificans, I trained my other leg, strengthened my upper body, and continued swimming. I refused to let the setback define me. When I finally returned, I came back stronger, dropping a tough opponent, Alex Martin, in the first round and winning a dominant unanimous decision. The time off wasn't wasted. It was an opportunity to build and enhance other areas of my game.

Finding New Ways to Improve

Injuries can feel like roadblocks, but they're actually opportunities in disguise. When you're forced to step back from your usual routine, you have time to focus on aspects of your game that you might have overlooked. Instead of dwelling on what you can't do, find what you can. A hand injury doesn't mean you stop training. It simply means you sharpen and improve other tools.

When I injured my hand, I focused on training the other, and before long, I was landing knockouts with what used to be my weaker side. Joe Calzaghe did the same thing. With injured hands, he adjusted his training, focusing on throwing fast, high-volume combinations instead of relying on power punches. His injury didn't limit him, it made him an even more dangerous fighter. This is the essence of determination. Finding every possible way to improve, no matter what the circumstance.

Maintaining a Healthy Lifestyle

Recovery doesn't end with physical therapy. It's about giving your body what it needs to heal. Proper nutrition, adequate rest, and a positive mindset. Eating the right foods, staying hydrated, and making sure you get enough sleep all contribute to a faster and stronger recovery. Your body heals while you rest, so make sleep a priority.

Mental Training and Visualization

Injuries offer the perfect chance to work on your mental game. Visualization can be a powerful tool. Mentally rehearsing your moves keeps your mind engaged and can even maintain your muscle memory. Picture yourself executing techniques perfectly, feeling every motion in your body. It's been proven that mental practice can help keep your skills sharp, even when you're not physically training.

Stay in love with learning. Watch footage, study your sport, and stay mentally ready for the moment your body is back to full strength. Just as your body needs conditioning, so does your mind.

Recover Smart, Not Fast

Patience is your best friend during recovery. Rushing back too soon can set you back further. Just like you'd follow a disciplined training routine, follow your rehab plan with the same focus. Slowly reintroduce stress to the injured area under the guidance of your team. Consistency is key here. Recovery is a process, and cutting corners can lead to longer-term damage.

Turning Losses into Lessons

> *"There is no losing in boxing. Either you win or you learn."* [38] —Lennox Lewis

Just like injuries, losses can teach you more than wins ever will. If you take the time to analyze what went wrong, you'll uncover areas that need improvement. Sugar Ray Robinson, one of the greatest boxers ever, didn't have a perfect record. His losses made him better. Bernard Hopkins, another legend, lost his first professional fight but went on to defend his title 20 times. His losses weren't setbacks, they were launchpads for greatness. In fact, for many athletes, setbacks become the very reason they are driven to reach new heights. These moments can fuel the fire that pushes you to improve and become unstoppable.

After taking a close loss to former world champion Luis Collazo, I refused to let it define me. He was a crafty veteran, coming off a brutal knockout win over a highly touted undefeated prospect. We went toe to toe in a war, and he edged me out in a majority decision. Instead of dwelling on it, I doubled down on my training, built a stronger team, and came back to beat former champion Breidis Prescott and stop Domonique Dolton, a dangerous fighter from the legendary Kronk Gym—in the third

---

[38] Lewis, Lennox. Interview following his 2001 rematch victory over Hasim Rahman, discussing his approach to setbacks and victories in boxing.

round. That loss to Collazo wasn't the end of anything. It was the moment that made me level up.

Setbacks like these teach resilience, grit, and the value of perseverance. In boxing, just as in life, setbacks are temporary, but the lessons they teach are permanent. Losses and injuries shape your mental fortitude, giving you the strength to push forward even when things don't go your way. They challenge you to grow, to adapt, and to keep moving forward no matter the obstacles.

Moving Forward

Injuries and losses are part of the game. How you respond is what makes the difference. Accept the injury, adapt your training, stay positive, and keep moving forward. Every setback is a stepping stone, and if you're willing to learn and grow from it, there's no limit to how far you can go.

Remember, challenges are temporary, but the lessons you learn will stay with you for life. Constantly pursue improvement and let each obstacle push you closer to becoming the best version of yourself, both in and out of the ring.

Chapter 20
Excellence in Preparation: Striving for Elite Status

"If you stay ready, you won't have to get ready." [39]

By the time the bell rings, the fight is already won or lost in the preparation that came before it.

In boxing, *preparation is everything.* Opportunities in the ring come and go in a split second. If you're not ready when they appear, they'll slip through your fingers, and so will your chance at winning. As the saying goes, "Success happens when preparation meets opportunity." The work you put in before the fight—your training, conditioning, nutrition and mindset—ensures that when the moment comes, you're ready to capitalize on it.

> *"I won the fight once the contract was signed."* [40] —Sugar Ray Robinson

This saying is a strong reminder that cutting corners in your training leads to disappointment. Just like a house without a solid foundation will collapse, a boxer who skips preparation will struggle when the pressure is on, no matter how "confident" he is.

Components of Preparation

Preparation involves several key areas:

Physical Conditioning: Your body needs to be in top shape to handle the demands of a fight. Regular, intense workouts build strength, speed, endurance, and agility. Every run, strength

---

[39] Traditional training maxim, popularized in combat sports and athletic preparation.

[40] Robinson, Sugar Ray. (Attributed quote). Widely cited quote reflecting his confidence in his preparation and training regimen. Robinson was a five-division world champion considered by many to be the greatest pound-for-pound boxer of all time.

workout, and heavy bag session gets you closer to peak physical readiness.

Technical Skill Development: Perfecting your technique takes time and practice. Hours spent drilling, shadowboxing, and working with partners ensure your punches, footwork, and defense become second nature. The sharper your technique, the more effective you'll be in the ring.

Mental Fortitude: Mental conditioning is just as important as physical training. Techniques like visualization, meditation, and mental rehearsals build the mental strength needed to stay calm and focused under pressure. A strong mind can elevate a good fighter to greatness.

Strategic Planning: Every opponent is unique, so preparation includes studying their habits, strengths, and weaknesses. Watching fight footage and analyzing their style helps you develop a game plan to exploit their vulnerabilities. NBA legend Kobe Bryant was famous for his obsessive study of opponents. He would watch hours of game footage, even picking apart players' tendencies to create the perfect strategy. Similarly, George St-Pierre, a dominant UFC champion, used detailed film study to break down his opponents' techniques and tendencies, allowing him to capitalize on their weaknesses. Boxers must adopt this same level of dedication to strategic planning, tailoring their approach to each opponent.

Nutrition and Recovery: What you put into your body and how well you rest are just as important as training. A balanced diet, proper hydration, and enough rest ensure your body performs at its best and recovers from tough workouts.

Levels of Excellence

To illustrate the importance of preparation, consider the following table that outlines the different levels of excellence:

Here, "Champion" refers to fighters who've earned a title—no small feat, but may not yet consistently dominate or evolve beyond their opposition.

Achieving elite status in preparation means excelling in every part of your training, including mindset. It's about pushing yourself to reach the next level. By doing this, you're doing more than just getting ready for your fight. You're preparing to dominate.

Every tough workout, round of training, and disciplined action you take is like depositing into your physical bank account. The more you invest, the more you can withdraw on fight night.

Failure to Prepare is Preparing to Fail

Preparation is the foundation of success in the ring. It's about consistently putting in effort, discipline, and determination to build your skill and toughness. When the moment comes, those who've prepared well will be ready to succeed, while those who haven't will struggle. Every minute spent preparing brings you closer to victory. Put in the work, make those deposits, and be ready to cash in when it matters most.

Practical Tips

Set Clear Goals: Know what you want to accomplish in each training session. For example, in a heavy bag session, your goal might be to maintain a steady pace for all rounds, focusing on proper form, balance, and power without fatigue breaking down your technique. For footwork practice, you could aim to complete five rounds of controlled lateral movement drills without crossing your feet. If you're sparring, a goal could be to land that specific counterpunch you've been working on.

Track Your Progress: Use a training journal (a free downloadable template is available at bryantperrella.com) to keep an eye on your progress and spot areas for improvement. Measure progress by tracking key areas like:

Sparring: Are you getting hit less? Are you landing more clean shots? Are you maintaining composure under pressure?

Skill Work: Are your combinations flowing smoother? Are you executing defensive movements instinctively?

Strength & Conditioning: Is your roadwork getting easier? Are your sprint times improving? Are you lifting heavier or doing more reps with ease?

Stay Consistent: Consistency is crucial. Regular training is the foundation for success. A solid weekly structure for a boxer could include sparring once or twice a week, skill work at least three-four times per week, strength training twice per week, and conditioning (cardio) around four times per week. Adjust based on your recovery and fight schedule.

Commit to the Process: Understand that preparation takes time. Accept the daily hard work as part of your journey to reaching the top. Boxing is about accumulation. Every round, every rep, and every session builds towards mastery.

Level	Psychological (Mindset)	Physical (Fitness/ Strength)	Technical (Proper Mechanics)	Tactical (Game Strategy)
Prospect	Good	Good	Good	Good
Champion	Better	Better	Better	Better
Elite	Best	Best	Best	Best

Round 4: Training Blueprint

Chapter 21
Training Camp: The Blueprint for Fight Readiness

"Victorious warriors win first and then go to war, while defeated warriors go to war first and then seek to win." [41]
—Sun Tzu

For generations, training camp has been the backbone of fight preparation, especially for old-school fighters who would isolate themselves, moving away from distractions to focus solely on the fight ahead. Legends of the past knew that a fight was won long before stepping into the ring. It was forged in the weeks of brutal, disciplined training, where the only priorities were eating, sleeping, and breathing boxing. Some fighters still follow this tradition by traveling to a separate location for camp, often to high-altitude areas or secluded environments that minimize distractions. Others choose to stay at their home gym, structuring their camp within familiar surroundings. There are also well-established training camps where fighters can train alongside top-notch boxers, gaining access to top-tier coaching, sparring, and resources.

Regardless, the moment a fighter enters training camp, the message is clear: this is serious business. Every decision from that point forward is made with one goal in mind—showing up in peak condition, mentally and physically, on the day of the fight.

The gloves feel heavier with every punch. Your arms burn, your legs ache, and your chest heaves with every breath. Your opponent, relentless, pressing forward without hesitation, stalks you. You've already pushed through round after round, but your coach calls for one more.

---

[41] Sun Tzu. *The Art of War.* Chapter 4: Tactical Dispositions. Translated by Lionel Giles, 1910. Written circa 5th century BCE.

This is where fights are won. Not under the bright lights, not in front of the crowd, but here, in the trenches... where the truth shows itself, and transformation takes place.

Fighters don't rise to the occasion, they fall to their level of their preparation.

Training camp is not exclusively about sharpening your skills. It's about pushing past your limits when fatigue has stolen your speed, when your body is begging for a break. One more round. One more rep. One more step forward when every part of you wants to step back. The fighter who leaves camp the most prepared is ahead of his opponent before the first punch is even thrown.

What Is a Training Camp?

A training camp is a structured, high-intensity preparation period before a fight, typically lasting six to 12 weeks. It is designed to bring a fighter to peak performance by focusing on conditioning, skill refinement, fight strategy, and weight management while ensuring recovery and mental sharpness leading into fight night.

Training camps follow a structured progression, but the specifics of workload, volume, and intensity are covered in the chapter on periodization later in the book.

How It Works

A standard training camp includes:

Skill Work: Shadowboxing, mitt work, bag drills, and sparring.

Conditioning: Roadwork, interval training and explosive strength training.

Strategy Development: Watching film, drilling setups, and working on opponent-specific tactics.

Recovery & Nutrition: Sleep, mobility work, physiotherapy, and proper fueling for weight cut.

Each session is carefully planned to maximize performance while preventing burnout, ensuring that the fighter peaks at the right time for fight night.

Who's Involved in a Training Camp?

At the elite level, fighters often have a full team of specialists, each focusing on different aspects of preparation. However, a successful training camp doesn't require every one of these roles. It depends on structured, quality work and making the most of available resources.

A training camp may include:

Head Coach: The foundation of any camp, overseeing overall training and fight strategy.

Assistant Coaches/Trainers: May specialize in areas such as defense, footwork, counterpunching, or specific fight strategies.

Sparring Partners: Essential for real fight preparation and simulating different styles. Some fighters bring in multiple sparring partners to mimic their upcoming opponent's style, while others rely on their gym's stable of fighters.

Strength & Conditioning Coach: Helps improve endurance, explosiveness, and injury prevention.

Nutritionist/Dietitian: Manages weight cut and fueling strategies, though many fighters handle this themselves.

Physiotherapist/Massage Therapist: Supports recovery, mobility, and injury prevention.

Sports Psychologist/Mental Coach: Helps with mindset, handling pressure, and mental resilience, though not all fighters utilize one.

The Structure of a Training Camp Varies

Some fighters train at one dedicated location with a full team in-house, while others piece together their preparation by training at different gyms for boxing, strength work, and sparring. Many fighters don't have access to a full team and instead work with what's available: whether it's handling their own strength and conditioning, training across multiple gyms, or relying on experienced coaches who take on multiple roles. The key isn't having the "perfect" setup. It is about maximizing the resources at hand and structuring camp for peak effectiveness.

Why Training Camp Is Important

Without a structured training camp, a fighter risks:

- Diminished conditioning and fatigue in the later rounds.
- Slower timing and less precision in execution.
- Difficulty adjusting in the fight or following a strategic game plan.
- Peaking too early, overtraining, or arriving flat by fight night.

A well-planned camp ensures that by the day of the fight, a fighter is physically and mentally ready, with their game plan drilled into their mind and conditioning dialed in.

Example: Full-Time Fighter's Training Camp Schedule (6 to 12 Weeks Out)

Morning (10:00 AM-11:30 AM): Boxing Training (mitt work, bag drills, footwork, tactical drills, light sparring).

Afternoon (2:00 PM-3:00 PM): Strength & Conditioning (explosive power, injury prevention, mobility work).

Evening (8:00 PM-9:00 PM): Roadwork (4-5 miles steady-state OR interval sprints/hill runs).

Sparring Days: Sparring generally replaces technical boxing on select days (e.g., two or three times per week) to allow proper recovery.

Recovery Focus: Hydration, stretching, physiotherapy, nutrition optimization, and quality sleep.

Note: Session times can be adjusted based on the flow of camp, fighter recovery, and specific training goals. Some fighters may shift roadwork to mornings or adjust sparring frequency based on how their body responds throughout camp.

How to Structure a Training Camp If You Have a Full-Time Job

Some fighters balance full-time jobs while training for a fight. While the structure remains the same, time management becomes key.

Training Structure For Fighters Balancing Work & Life Obligations:

Morning (30-45 minutes): Roadwork (steady-state running, interval sprints, or hill sprints).

Evening (60-90 minutes): Boxing Training + Strength & Conditioning (mitt work, bag drills, sparring, explosive strength work).

Strength Training: 2-3 three times per week, focusing on power, injury prevention, and explosive movements.

Weekend Sparring: Prioritize hard rounds when time allows.

Getting the most from each session:

> **High-intensity, focused sessions** over long, drawn-out training.

> **Prioritizing recovery** (hydration, sleep, and mobility work).

> **Strategic drilling** to develop clean, reliable execution instead of excessive bag work.

Even with limited time, a structured camp puts a fighter in position to arrive in peak condition without overtraining or burning out.

Chapter 22
Getting Fit to Fight

"The fight is won or lost in the preparation long before the fight starts."[42]—Joe Louis

Every action you take or do not take ultimately leads to your level of physicality.

Beyond strength and stamina, true physicality is about a commanding aura. It is an intangible presence. It radiates from the fighter who has put in the work. It shows in the way they move, how they maintain their composure, and how they control the fight, moment by moment. It's something that can't be faked or forced. It's earned through hard work, sacrifice, and repetition. And when it's earned, you feel it. You carry it with you into the ring, where it seeps through every step, every punch, and every breath. Physicality is the fusion of skill, conditioning, and confidence, where mastery of technique, endurance, and control allows a fighter to dictate the fight and impose their will.

As we've mentioned earlier, mindset plays a critical role in a warrior's journey. Achieving a true state of confidence requires belief in your abilities, cultivated through preparation and experience. However, to suggest that boxing is mainly mental overlooks a vital truth: physical and mental strength are deeply intertwined. Confidence and belief mean little if you're not in top physical condition. Without the fitness, endurance, and power to back up your mental resolve, confidence becomes a façade, an illusion that shatters under pressure. Ultimately, your body's capability determines your limits. If you step into the ring physically outmatched, no amount of mental fortitude can compensate for the gap. You'll find yourself struggling to keep up, falling back on your physical capacity...or lack thereof.

---

[42] Louis, Joe, (Attributed quote). Former Heavyweight Champion who held the title for 11 years and 8 months (1937-1949), the longest reign in heavyweight history with 25 successful title defenses.

This relationship between physical and mental prowess is inseparable. Physical conditioning fuels your mentality, instilling a sense of power that translates into a confident and dominant presence. When your body is strong, your mind follows suit, creating an unshakable combination. Simply put: you choose whether to be predator or prey. Physicality bleeds into your mindset, helping you embody the conqueror's spirit. With that being said, let's get into it.

Having greater physical ability than your opponent gives you a tremendous advantage. Imagine having more strength, power, punch resistance, and stamina than your opponent in a video game. They'll tire out faster because they have to push harder to keep up, while you remain composed, operating well within your capacity.

The truth is, all elite fighters express their physicality in the ring, though it leans in different directions. Some fighters, like Rocky Marciano, Evander Holyfield, and Artur Beterbiev, blend power, pressure, and relentless endurance, breaking opponents down with intelligent aggression and unshakable will. Others, like Floyd Mayweather Jr., Sugar Ray Robinson, and Manny Pacquiao, express their athletic prowess through explosiveness, blistering speed, and fluid skill, weaving their athletic gifts seamlessly into their styles.

Being in the ring with a fighter like this feels like working with a heavier bag instead of a lighter one. It takes more out of you, even if the difference isn't obvious at first. Every movement, every punch from them feels deliberate and dense, like it carries extra weight. They don't need to force anything. Step by step, punch by punch, they drain your energy as you try to keep up.

How It Unfolds in the Ring

It's not what you do, it's how you do it. This control flows through every movement, every punch, every adjustment. Some fighters overwhelm their opponents with constant pressure, while others stay patient, quickly strike in and out of range, frustrating their opponents with explosive footwork and combinations. They always seem in control, one step ahead, and this is exhausting to deal with.

Endurance: This advantage shows in the later rounds, where others begin to fade. It's more than lasting longer. It's about staying calm and composed while your opponent, increasingly tense, expends more energy just to keep up. The deeper the fight goes, the more comfortable you become.

Speed and Execution: Speed is more than being fast, it's about using it with intent. Clean pivots and well-timed punches leave your opponent chasing, always a step behind. The more smoothly you move, the slower they seem.

Power with Precision: Power isn't in how hard you swing, it's how well you place it. One clean shot at the right time can shake confidence, flip momentum, and shift the entire fight.

Control and Balance: Control keeps you grounded, always ready to act or react. When your movements are purposeful, you dictate the pace, forcing your opponent to fight on your terms.

You Run the Show

When you've earned this presence, it becomes a kind of confidence, a quiet certainty that flows through every action. You don't need to force anything, because the fight unfolds on your terms. This sense of control weighs on your opponent with every movement. While they scramble to adjust, you stay calm, cool and calculated. When you're tired, they're exhausted. When they push harder, they only sink faster.

Boxing Training: The Best Form of Conditioning

> *"If there is one abiding theme in the gym, it's the withering work in the ring. Those not fit do not survive."* [43]—Emanuel Steward, renowned trainer

---

[43] Steward, Emanuel. Quote from "Boxing's Hall of Fame Trainer" interview, ESPN Boxing, 2008. Steward was the founder of Kronk Gym and trained over 40 world champions including Tommy Hearns, Lennox Lewis, and Wladimir Klitschko.

Many people misunderstand the best way to get in shape for boxing. Often, strength and conditioning or general fitness training is prioritized too heavily over actual boxing workouts. While these are important for building overall athleticism, the reality is much simpler: boxing should remain the central focus. It's where the majority of your time and energy should go. If you want to be in peak condition for a fight, boxing training needs to be of utmost priority, with strength and conditioning revolving around it.

Just look at the training routines of legendary boxers. Success leaves clues, and these champions didn't try to reinvent the wheel, they focused on intense, consistent boxing training. Of course, they also integrated conditioning to increase strength, power, and endurance. But ultimately, the most important factor in being fight-ready is the boxing training itself. Nothing beats the physical and mental conditioning that comes from focused boxing practice.

True boxing conditioning is more than being in shape, it's about sustaining technique and output under exhaustion. Skill work under fatigue is what prepares you for the later rounds, so your punches stay sharp even when your body wants to slow down. Hitting the bag, working mitts, or sparring when your arms are heavy and your legs are burning builds the fight-specific endurance no amount of general conditioning can replace.

Not only that, but the act of boxing itself is what sharpens your instincts, refines your technique, and increases your skills. Every round on the mitts, bag, or in sparring forces you to problem-solve in real time, adapt to different styles, and internalize movement patterns until they become second nature. Without this, no amount of conditioning or strength training will give you the tools needed to dominate in the ring.

Boxing rounds in training typically last three minutes with a one-minute rest in between, mimicking the conditions of an actual fight and building the stamina needed to perform at your best. However, to gain an edge, many fighters go beyond this.

They might extend the work periods to four or five minutes (or longer) and reduce the rest periods to 30 seconds or less.

Important: These kinds of extreme training demands, including extended rounds, shortened rest periods, and high-mileage running, are typically reserved for the peak of a training camp and are not maintained year-round.

Some fighters even do multiple boxing sessions in a single day to double down on what matters most. This strategy pushes both body and mind to their limits, boosting overall endurance for the ring.

Note for Amateurs: The following examples of training intensity reflect what world-class professionals do to reach elite levels. If you're just starting out or aren't fighting full-time, don't feel pressured to match these extremes. Focus on building a strong base, staying consistent, and progressing at your own pace. Use the principles here as inspiration, not obligation.

Also keep in mind: Recovery is just as important as the work itself. Overtraining without adequate rest can break your body down instead of building it up. For a deeper dive into recovery strategies, including sleep and nutrition, refer to Round 7.

Examples of Intense Training Regimens

The following are extreme examples from some of the best fighters in the world. Their training regimens reflect years of progression, discipline, and relentless work. But remember, you are your own competition. The goal isn't to match them today but to push your limits and increase your workload over time in a way that suits your own development.

Floyd Mayweather Jr.

Mayweather's training was built around extreme boxing volume with minimal rest. His workouts sometimes stretched over 30-40 total rounds, covering:

Sparring ("Doghouse Rules"): Sessions continued until someone quit, sometimes lasting 15 to 30 minutes straight, eliminating the safety of timed rounds and conditioning fighters to work through exhaustion.

Heavy Bag Work: Mayweather frequently went 30+ minutes non-stop, throwing fast, sharp combinations.

Mitt Work: High-speed defensive drills focused on hand speed, reflexes, and technical sharpness. He often did long, uninterrupted rounds with his trainer and uncle, two-weight world champion Roger Mayweather, reinforcing his signature defensive movements.

Body Shield Drills: Intense body shield work, where he hammered hooks, uppercuts, and jabs to the midsection for 10+ minutes straight. Building punching endurance and ensuring power remained consistent deep into fights.

Speed Bag & Double-End Bag: Sharpening rhythm, timing, hand-eye coordination, and arm endurance.

Shadowboxing: Often performed at the start of training, sometimes with light hand weights to build shoulder endurance and punching stamina.

Ankle Weight Training: Mayweather has also trained with ankle weights during boxing and jump rope sessions to develop lower body strength and agility.

Additional Conditioning

Jump Rope: High-intensity jump rope sessions for foot speed and rhythm.

Running: 5-8+ miles daily (in camp), maintaining a steady pace for endurance.

Pool Work: Has implemented swimming into his routine to improve cardiovascular fitness and overall conditioning.

Mayweather only pauses for a sip of water before jumping into the next round, mimicking the endurance needed to stay sharp for 12+ full rounds.

Errol Spence Jr.

Famous for grueling long boxing sessions with minimal breaks. Spence is known for his relentless pressure, consistent power, and a high-volume attack. His ability to maintain his work rate is built through high-volume boxing training and additional strength-endurance work.

Sparring: 19 consecutive rounds confirmed. Sometimes over 20 in a single session during training camp. He spars with fresh partners rotating in, forcing him to stay sharp under fatigue.

Heavy Bag Work: 15+ rounds, focusing on constant pressure and sustained punching to simulate his high-output style.

Mitt Work: Part of extended, high-intensity boxing sessions punching over 45+ minutes straight with minimal breaks. Spence works on punch placement, inside fighting, and countering pressure, maintaining a steady pace throughout.

Body Work Drills: Hundreds of hard, thudding body shots thrown per session, reinforcing his signature liver shots and building endurance in his punching muscles.

Technical Drills: Repeated drills focusing on punch placement and balance, ensuring every shot carries power even when fatigued.

Additional Conditioning

Calisthenics (High-Volume Bodyweight Training): Push-ups, pull-ups, dips, and ab work to build strength-endurance, allowing him to punch consistently with power late into fights.

Running: 5-6 miles at a fast pace, reinforcing his ability to keep pushing forward without slowing down.

Everything in Spence's training revolves around sustaining a relentless pace while keeping his shots heavy and damaging.

Terence "Bud" Crawford

Rigorous training routines that build incredible stamina and resilience.

Crawford's training is built on adaptability, pace shifts, and an ability to finish stronger than his opponents. His high-altitude training and intense circuit-style boxing workouts give him elite endurance, mental toughness, and a late-fight edge.

Sparring: Crawford regularly spars top-level fighters, including Shakur Stevenson and Andre Ward, pushing himself against elite competition. His sparring sessions emphasize a relentless work rate, conditioning him to stay sharp under fatigue and maintain his edge deep into fights.

5+ Minute Rounds Instead of 3: To simulate championship fight conditions, Crawford often spars and trains in longer-than-standard rounds with short rest periods.

90-Minute Non-Stop Circuit Workouts: Crawford has done non-stop training sessions, transitioning between:

- **Mitt Work:** Rounds focusing on speed and precision.
- **Heavy Bag:** Extended rounds maintaining high output and power.
- **Double-End Bag:** Enhancing reflexes, timing, and accuracy while staying sharp under fatigue.
- **Jumping Exercises (on Tires):** Developing explosive endurance in the legs.
- **Stationary Bike Sprints:** Keeping heart rate elevated between boxing rounds.
- **Shadowboxing & Slipping Drills:** Active recovery while reinforcing defensive movement.
- **Body Work Focus:** Intense bodyshield punching to ensure power is sustained deep into fights.

Additional Conditioning

Altitude Training in Colorado Springs: Trains at 6,000+ feet elevation, forcing his body to become more efficient with oxygen use, leading to better endurance and faster recovery. His high-altitude regimen includes intense mountain runs and hikes, pushing his cardiovascular system to its limits.

Strength Work & Conditioning: Includes explosive med-ball throws, bodyweight exercises, weight training, and agility drills to reinforce his power and mobility. Along with traditional strength training, he incorporates swimming and other cross-training methods, making him one of the most well-rounded athletes in the sport. All of this further enhances his physicality, allowing him to impose his presence in the ring.

Unpredictable Pace & Adaptability: Crawford's training is beyond endurance, it's about being fresh enough to adjust at any moment, break opponents mentally, and finish fights strong.

Note: Unlike circuits that alternate between short bursts of boxing and conditioning (e.g., 30 seconds boxing, 30 seconds circuit exercise), Crawford's 90-minute non-stop session emphasizes sustained rounds of boxing work before switching to the next station. This means he's getting the full effect of real fight pacing—spending at least three minutes or more per modality—before transitioning to another exercise while staying in motion.

Fight-Specific Adaptations Matter

Training your body to sustain work for full rounds is key to boxing conditioning. Constantly switching quickly between different exercises, like doing 30 seconds of jumping jacks, then 30 seconds on the heavy bag, followed by 30 seconds of push-ups, **doesn't simulate the actual demands of a fight**. It conditions your body to expect breaks and different movements. True boxing endurance comes from pushing through full-length rounds of actual boxing work, just as you will in the ring.

That being said, short-interval circuits do have value for general fitness. These quick-switch workouts can be great for boosting your overall athleticism, cardiovascular endurance, and explosive output. They may also help beginners build a base level of conditioning before transitioning into full boxing rounds. They can even be used as a hybrid session, combining boxing movements with muscular conditioning to add variety while reinforcing boxing-specific patterns under fatigue.

This approach can improve muscular endurance, sharpen focus under pressure, and help you maintain proper form when tired. However, for fighters preparing for competition, complete boxing rounds must take priority, because it builds the specific rhythm, timing, and mental toughness required for real rounds in the ring. You fight until the bell rings.

Why Boxing Comes First

Boxing training is the foundation. It builds the specific endurance, movement, and fight conditioning needed in the ring. From there, additional work like cardio further develops stamina, while strength and conditioning enhances overall power and resilience. Each element plays a role, but everything revolves around boxing first.

Hence, we will begin by explaining the main tools that fighters have at their disposal, setting the foundation for what follows.

To further reinforce this, we'll now break down the science behind why boxing-specific training is the cornerstone of fight conditioning and the key to preparing for real competition.

The SAID Principle: The Fighter's Edge

> *"The body adapts to the stress put upon it."* [44] —Hans Selye & Julius Wolff

Boxing places unique demands on both the body and mind, requiring a blend of high-intensity bursts of effort, precise

---

[44] Hans Selye and Julius Wolff were pioneers in stress physiology and biomechanics, respectively. Selye developed the General Adaptation Syndrome theory (1936), while Wolff is known for Wolff's Law (1892), which states that bone adapts to mechanical stress. This quote synthesizes their foundational ideas.

technique, quick reflexes, and strategic thinking under pressure. These demands can only be developed through training specifically tailored to the sport of boxing. This is where the SAID principle comes into play.

SAID stands for Specific Adaptation to Imposed Demands, meaning your body adapts directly to the type of training you do. By doing boxing-specific workouts, you're conditioning your body to handle the exact stresses you'll face in the ring, making you better equipped for real fights.

Boxing drills like shadowboxing, mitt work, heavy bag sessions, sparring, and using the double-end bag all improve key attributes such as endurance, strength, coordination, and mental toughness. Each of these exercises mirrors the demands of the sport, helping you build the fitness and skills that directly translate to better performance in the ring.

Skills Pay the Bills

At the highest level, fights aren't won by brute force or sheer endurance alone, they're won by skill. Not only does boxing training develop your conditioning, but it also hones your instincts, locks in your technique, and expands your repertoire of moves. Every round of shadowboxing, mitt work, or sparring forces you to make real-time adjustments, solve problems on the fly, and internalize movement patterns until they become second nature.

And skill isn't something you're born with, it's forged through endless repetition. The only way to truly develop it is by putting in the rounds, practicing each movement until it becomes automatic. Without this, no amount of conditioning or strength training will give you the tools needed to dominate in the ring. A well-trained fighter can dictate the pace, break opponents down systematically, and capitalize on openings quickly.

Strength, endurance, and power all play a role...but skills pay the bills.

The Role of Strength & Conditioning

Don't get it twisted. Strength training, running, and bodyweight exercises are important for building the athletic qualities needed in boxing—like power, endurance, and resilience. These exercises complement your boxing training, enhancing your performance and helping you handle the physical demands of the ring.

If you want a complete breakdown of how to build strength, endurance, and explosive power as a fighter—from calisthenics to weightlifting to advanced methods—refer to Chapter 25: Building Your Machine. It's a full roadmap for developing the physical tools that back up your boxing skills.

However, while they offer important benefits, the training that best prepares you for competition is the work that reflects the realities of boxing itself. In the next sections, we'll explore how these elements come together to develop you as a complete fighter.

Shadowboxing: Crafting the Invisible Fight

Shadowboxing, or practicing your boxing movements (whether in front of a mirror, with a target in mind, or in open space while simulating an opponent), is a fundamental part of boxing training that sharpens your technique, improves footwork, and enhances your skills—all without the need for equipment or a partner. The mirror acts as a valuable tool to let you perfect your form and movements, building muscle memory and reflexes while developing your rhythm and flow. Without the mirror, shadowboxing becomes more about visualization and imagination. Picturing your opponent, anticipating reactions, and exploring movement freely.

Many champions consider shadowboxing one of the most important exercises in their routine. It allows you to visualize your opponent and mentally rehearse strategies. The beauty of shadowboxing is that it's only limited by your imagination. This is where your creativity can flow, allowing you to experiment with new movements and setups. This practice is essential for developing your skills, helping you anticipate and react faster when you're in the ring.

Benefits of Shadowboxing

Refine Techniques: Perfect your punches, defensive moves, and combinations.

Improve Footwork: Maintain balance and fluidity while moving.

Enhance Defensive Movement: Practice slipping, ducking, and weaving to avoid punches.

Develop Muscle Memory: Repetition ingrains movements into muscle memory for quicker reactions.

Boost Reflexes and Reaction Time: Sharpen your reflexes and improve your reaction time.

Work on Rhythm and Flow: Discover and maintain your unique rhythm during a fight.

Unleash Creativity: Shadowboxing lets your imagination run free, allowing you to explore new strategies and combinations.

Drills to Elevate Your Shadowboxing

Punching & Defensive Drills

Jab-Only Round: Spend a full round using only the jab, focusing on speed, accuracy, and different variations (e.g., double jab, feint-jab, stepping in and out).

Counter-Slip Drill: Simulate an opponent's jab, slip to the outside, and return with a counter right hand. Repeat while moving forward and backward.

Head Movement & Defense Focus: Perform a full round without throwing a punch, only slipping, rolling, parrying, and moving your head as if an opponent were attacking.

Fight Scenario Rounds: Visualize an opponent with a specific style (pressure fighter, counterpuncher, long-range boxer) and adjust your movement, counters, and strategy accordingly.

Finish Strong Round: In the last 30 seconds of a round, simulate an aggressive finish by increasing punch volume and movement, conditioning your mind and body to finish strong.

Footwork Drills

Step & Pivot Drill: Throw a combination, pivot out at an angle, then reset before throwing again. This reinforces sharp movement and positioning after punching.

Lateral Movement Round: Shadowbox using only side-to-side movement, focusing on circling, stepping off the centerline, and maintaining balance while moving laterally.

In-and-Out Drill: Step in with a punch or combination, then quickly step back out to simulate controlling distance and avoiding counters.

Quarter Turn Drill: After every 2-3 punches, take a slight quarter-turn step to practice repositioning and creating angles.

Cutting Off the Ring: Shadowbox while imagining an opponent moving away. Cut off their space using controlled lateral steps while keeping pressure.

Pressure Response Drill: Shadowbox while imagining a pressure fighter coming forward. Practice stepping back, countering, and angling off. This helps build comfort under pressure and teaches you how to reset your position and control distance without getting trapped.

Mitt Work: Building the Fighter's Toolbox

Mitt work, or working on punching techniques with a trainer using pads, is a key part of boxing training that goes beyond just throwing punches. It's a hands-on and dynamic routine that builds skills, strategies, and mental toughness, while also strengthening the boxing connection between you and your trainer.

Learning from Your Trainer

One of the main advantages of mitt work is learning from your trainer's knowledge and experience. As they call out combinations, defensive moves, and counterpunches, you have to quickly react and follow through. Unlike hitting a heavy bag, mitt work improves the mind-muscle connection because you're working with a live person. You're not just punching, you're blocking, slipping, and rolling with someone in front of you. This real-time interaction boosts your timing, accuracy, and defense, making these movements second nature over time. Trainers may also use tools like the power shield and body shield during mitt work to help you practice landing powerful punches or deliver hard body shots safely while maintaining proper form.

Building a Connection

Mitt work helps strengthen the understanding between you and your trainer or coach. During these sessions, your trainer gets to know your strengths and weaknesses, giving you real-time feedback to help you improve. In return, you learn to trust their guidance and respond quickly under pressure. This close partnership is indispensable in pushing you to reach your full potential, both in training and in the ring.

Increases Endurance

Mitt work goes beyond technique, it also builds serious endurance. Unlike bag work or shadowboxing, where you set your own pace, mitt work forces you to match your trainer's rhythm. Even when you're tired, you have to maintain intensity and fire off quick combinations. This constant pace pushes your physical limits and mimics the kind of sustained output you'll need in a real fight.

It also forces you to stay sharp on defense when you're tired. You're blocking, slipping, and staying aware, even when fatigue sets in. This is crucial in real fights, where being alert and protecting yourself is important, especially in the later rounds. By pushing through that exhaustion, you build the stamina and mental toughness needed to perform at your best, even when your gas tank is running low.

Improving Technique

Mitt work is the perfect way to sharpen your technique. Your trainer can quickly point out and correct any mistakes, helping you adjust your punches and movements right away. This instant feedback ensures you're using the right form and getting the most out of your performance. Whether you're working on combinations, defense, or power, mitt work helps you improve and grow as a fighter.

Developing Defensive Skills

Mitt work also boosts your defense. Your trainer can mimic different attacks, letting you practice dodging, slipping, and countering in real time. This builds your reflexes and teaches you to stay composed under pressure, getting you ready for the unexpected in real fights.

Working with Different Pad Holders

While your main trainer may hold mitts for you most of the time, working with different pad holders can introduce new techniques and perspectives. Each trainer has their own style, and learning from multiple sources can make you a more adaptable and well-rounded fighter.

Heavy Bag: Unleash Your Power

Heavy bag training is the go-to for building both power and endurance. Hitting the bag with proper form simulates the impact of a real fight and also increases your punching strength. The heavy bag's dense resistance absorbs your energy, pushing your body to work harder, which boosts both your power and stamina. As you keep hitting the bag, you're learning to punch harder, you're also conditioning your body to sustain energy and strength through multiple rounds.

Different Approaches to Heavy Bag Training

There are a few key methods to approaching heavy bag training, each with its own focus:

Hit and Move: You can treat the bag like a moving opponent, practicing footwork and throwing punches while in motion. This approach builds agility and increases your ability to strike effectively while moving around the ring.

Stationary Power: Some boxers focus on standing still and throwing strong, powerful punches. This method helps you concentrate on generating as much force as possible with each punch, which can build knockout power.

Combination of Both: A versatile approach is to mix movement with powerful combinations. Move around the bag like it's an opponent, then stop to deliver heavy punches. This blend improves both your movement and power, making you adaptable in the ring.

Bag Drills

Adding specific drills to your heavy bag workouts can increase your conditioning and get you ready for different fight situations. Here are a few drills to try:

Intervals: Throw straight punches on the bag nonstop for 30 seconds, concentrating on output and "the burn". Then, spend the next 30 seconds moving around the bag throwing quick, lighter punches. This alternating cycle builds both punch endurance and boxing ability.

Power and Movement: Alternate between 30 seconds of sharp movement and quick combinations, then 30 seconds of planting your feet and unleashing full-power punches. This drill is designed to help you develop explosive punching power while transitioning smoothly between mobility and raw force.

Combination Repetition: Pick a specific combination, like jab-cross-hook or uppercut-hook-cross, and practice it repeatedly for a set time. You can do this solo or with a trainer using mitts or a noodle to keep you focused on defense between combinations. This drill helps improve your precision, speed, and defensive responsibility as you tire.

Fight Simulation Round: Set a timer for three-minute rounds. Start by moving around the bag, throwing combinations for one minute. Then, spend one minute standing still, focusing on heavy power punches. Finish the round with one minute of nonstop punching. This drill mimics the varied pace of a real fight and builds the strength needed to maintain power in later rounds.

George Foreman's Gruesome Heavy Bag Sessions

George Foreman, one of the most powerful punchers in boxing history, was notorious for his intense heavy bag sessions. He was known to punch deep indentations into the bag, a testament to his incredible strength and power. He would go an hour straight on the heavy bag, and at times during the session, he would focus on throwing only lefts, then only rights, and also go non-stop with both hands. These gruesome sessions were a key part of his training regimen, helping him develop the devastating punching power that made him a feared opponent in the ring. Foreman's ability to leave such marks on the heavy bag is a reminder of the potential in building immense strength and power with this method.

Benefits of Heavy Bag Training

The heavy bag is a key tool for improving various aspects of your boxing skills:

Strength Endurance: Repeatedly hitting the bag builds endurance in your arms, shoulders, and core. This helps you maintain power and technique throughout the fight.

Power: Each punch on the bag increases your raw punching power. With consistent practice, you'll notice a big improvement in the force of your punches.

Conditioning: Heavy bag workouts are intense and give you a great cardio workout. They boost your overall fitness, helping you stay in shape and keep your energy up during fights.

Technique: Regular heavy bag sessions allow you to improve your punching form, and work on combinations in a controlled setting.

The heavy bag will help you become a more powerful, well-conditioned fighter. Point blank, period.

Sparring: The Ultimate Test

"The bag doesn't hit back." [45]

Sparring is the ultimate test of your skills and abilities. Unlike the heavy bag, which can't hit back, sparring gives you a live, reactive opponent. It's where you can apply the techniques you've learned and test them in a controlled but realistic environment. During sparring sessions, you get a chance to work on your timing, footwork, defense, and offense in real time against an opponent. The ability to perform under pressure and think on your feet is critical in a boxing match, and sparring helps you develop those skills.

Sparring inside your gym doesn't always have to be a war. The key is making sure it's controlled. In-house sparring should be

---

[45] Traditional boxing maxim, popularized by Bruce Lee in "Enter the Dragon" (1973), commonly used in combat sports training to emphasize the difference between practice and real fighting.

monitored closely by coaches to ensure both fighters are improving, not simply trading damage. There's a time and place to go to war, and there's a time to sharpen weapons without dulling the edge.

The Benefits of Sparring

Realistic Practice: Sparring closely mimics an actual fight, giving you a chance to practice techniques in a more unpredictable environment. This helps prepare you mentally and physically for competition.

Developing Reflexes: Regular sparring sharpens your reflexes and quickens your reaction time. The constant movement and punches teach you to react naturally to your opponent's actions over time.

Enhancing Adaptability: Every sparring partner offers new challenges. Facing different styles helps you quickly adapt, a key skill for dealing with various opponents in real fights.

Building Endurance: Sparring is the ultimate test of endurance because it's the closest you'll get to the intensity of an actual fight. The fast pace and high intensity push your stamina to the limit, building the cardiovascular endurance you need to maintain your energy and strength throughout a match.

Mental Toughness: Sparring builds mental resilience, teaching you to stay calm under pressure, manage stress, and stay focused—skills essential for peak performance in the ring.

Defense Development: Another valuable tactic is sparring with fighters who have less experience than you. This allows you to focus on specific defensive movements repetitively in a lower-risk setting, sharpening your timing and reactions without the same pressure or danger as sparring high-level opponents. Training this way helps build instinctive defensive habits that you can later apply against more skilled fighters, where mistakes cost more. These sessions give you the space to stay composed, stay defensively responsible, and refine your awareness through consistent reps.

Evaluating Progress: It's a great way to track your progress. Sparring reveals both strengths to build on and weaknesses to work on, helping guide your training. Going out of your comfort zone and sparring in other competitive gyms, against new fighters, can help you become more accustomed to the pre-fight jitters and emotions you'll feel on fight night. Always sparring the same people won't fully prepare you, mentally or physically, for the unpredictability of a real opponent. Having others around watching as you spar can also help with this, since there will be eyes on you when you compete. Working closely with your coach during sparring helps you identify what to focus on, track your progress, and avoid falling into bad habits.

Strategic Thinking: Sparring also sharpens your mind. It helps you learn to anticipate moves, set traps, and think tactically—skills that can be applied in actual fights.

Types of Sparring

Combat Drills: Focuses on specific skills and techniques at a lighter intensity. It's great for working on particular aspects of your game without the full pressure of a hard sparring session. These drills help you practice key moves for fight night while minimizing the risk of injury.

Situational Sparring: Focuses on practicing in specific situations, like being stuck in a corner or facing a taller opponent. It helps prepare you for particular challenges you might encounter in a match.

Full-Contact Sparring: This is the most intense type of sparring, simulating an actual fight with full power and energy. It's non-negotiable for testing your skills under realistic conditions and building the endurance and toughness needed for a real match.

Combat Drills: Fine-Tuning Your Fight Game

"Drillers make killers." [46]

Combat drills are great for dialing in specific techniques without the intensity of full sparring. In these lighter sessions with a partner, the goal isn't to win but to work on certain areas of your game.

The Purpose of Combat Drills

Technical Mastery: Combat drills help you zero in on specific skills in a controlled environment. Whether it's your jab, defensive moves, or counter-punches, these drills give you the repetition needed to make those skills second nature.

Real-Time Application: While heavy bag work and shadowboxing are helpful, there's nothing like practicing moves on a live partner. Combat drills bridge the gap between solo practice and sparring by offering a more realistic setting to apply your techniques.

Muscle Memory: Repeating specific movements in a live drill helps your body memorize the motions much faster, making them automatic during sparring or real fights.

Quicker Reaction Time: Combat drills simulate different scenarios, allowing you to improve your reflexes and reaction time so you're prepared for a variety of situations in the ring.

Preserving the Fighter: Combat drills are lighter in intensity, which helps you stay fresh and healthy while still practicing realistic fight scenarios and preparing for fight night. While not the same as sparring, they offer a controlled way to develop sharp reactions and defensive instincts, much like how sparring with less experienced fighters can be used strategically to isolate and refine defensive movements without high risk.

---

[46] Common training maxim in combat sports, emphasizing that consistent drilling and repetition of techniques leads to fighting excellence. Origin uncertain.

Examples of Combat Drills

Catch-Counter Drill: One partner throws a set combination, and the other responds with counter punches. This drill helps both fighters work on their offense, defense, and counter-punching skills at the same time.

Body Shots Only Drill: In this drill, both fighters spar with the rule that only body shots are allowed, no headshots. It focuses on improving body-targeting accuracy, strengthening your defense, and amplifying your ability to counter body attacks.

Lead Hand Only Drill: Each fighter can only use their front hand, using jabs, hooks, and other lead hand techniques. This drill develops the lead hand's effectiveness and improves defensive skills related to the lead hand.

Controlled Defensive Flow Drill: One fighter applies light, continuous pressure with controlled punches while the other focuses purely on defense, working on slipping, parrying, blocking, and angling out without firing back. This helps refine defensive instincts, improve reaction time, and build confidence under pressure without taking unnecessary damage.

Success Through Combat Drills

Cuba and countries that were part of the former Soviet system have been powerhouses in amateur boxing, largely thanks to their emphasis on combat drills. Their approach focuses on structured, repetitive training, which fine-tunes technical skills and builds great awareness early in a boxer's career. This has been a key factor in their lasting success.

Bringing these same methods into your own routine can give you a big advantage. Combat drills help you tighten up your techniques, improve reaction time, and deepen your boxing knowledge. Combined with regular sparring, these drills will shape you into a more skilled and dangerous fighter in the ring.

Speed Bag: The Symphony of Skill

The speed bag is a timeless part of boxing training, used for generations, and for good reason. It's an effective tool for improving hand-eye coordination, rhythm, and timing. This small bag, hung from a platform, is struck with rapid punches, building hand speed and arm endurance to help you stay strong through the later rounds of a fight.

Benefits of Speed Bag Training

Improves Hand-Eye Coordination: It helps your brain and body work together to hit your target effectively.

Builds Arm Endurance: It strengthens your ability to maintain effective punches throughout the fight.

Strengthens Smaller Muscles: Often ignored, these muscles support punching speed and consistency over time.

Jump Rope: Skipping Your Way to Victory

Jump rope isn't child's play. It's one of the most valuable exercises for boxers, helping build footwork, coordination, and endurance. (You're simply hopping over the rope with rhythm, either on both feet or alternating. Done properly, it becomes a rhythmic dance of precision and speed.) In the ring, these skills are necessary for quick movements, delivering punches, dodging attacks, and maintaining balance.

Boxing greats like Sugar Ray Leonard and Roberto Duran were known for their incredible jump rope skills. Leonard's lightning-fast footwork and graceful movements were honed through his jump rope drills, contributing to his agility in the ring. Duran took it to another level, incorporating squatted jump rope variations to build strength and endurance in his legs. Their commitment to jump rope training highlights how crucial it is developing this skill, helping to succeed in boxing.

Benefits of Jump Rope Training

Improves Footwork: Jump rope drills help develop quick, agile movements, allowing boxers to move efficiently and stay light on their feet in the ring.

Builds Leg Strength: This exercise strengthens leg muscles, contributing to the power behind punches and providing the stability needed to hold your ground during a fight.

Increases Endurance: Jumping rope boosts lung capacity and overall stamina, keeping you energized and able to maintain your intensity throughout each round.

Develops Coordination: It increases your balance and control, improving how your body moves together and preparing you for executing more advanced techniques.

Jump rope can be used both at the beginning of a boxing session to warm up your muscles and get your blood flowing or at the end as a high-intensity finisher to push your endurance to the limit.

This straightforward yet powerful exercise is a staple in boxing, laying the groundwork for success in the ring.

Double-End Bag: Precision and Timing

Training with the double-end bag is like playing a fast-paced game of precision and timing. It's a great modality for enhancing hand-eye coordination, accuracy, and reflexes. This small, fast-moving target mimics an opponent's head movement, making it an amazing tool for sharpening your skills.

Roy Jones Jr., one of boxing's all-time greats, is renowned for his incredible skills on the double-end bag. This piece of equipment is one of his favorites, and he has perfected it to a level unseen. Watching Jones work the double-end bag is like witnessing a master at play, effortlessly combining speed, precision, and timing to stay many steps ahead of his opponents.

Benefits of Double-End Bag Training

Targets Punching Accuracy: Trains you to hit a moving target with precision, helping you land cleaner shots in real exchanges.

Improves Rhythm and Timing: Develops your ability to sense openings and react with the right punch at the right time.

Improves Hand-Eye Coordination: Teaches your hands and eyes to sync under pressure, so you can handle fast-paced combinations.

Increases Speed and Reflexes: Conditions your body to respond quicker—whether slipping, countering, or letting your hands go.

Additional Training Tools

Cobra Reflex Bag: A free-standing, spring-loaded bag that snaps back rapidly when hit, mimicking an opponent's counterpunch. It helps develop hand speed, precision, reaction time, and defensive reflexes. Fighters like Ryan Garcia use this tool to train their ability to strike quickly while staying alert and ready to avoid incoming shots.

Spar Bar: A rotating horizontal bar mounted on a central pole that swings back and forth when struck. It sharpens reflexes and reinforces defensive habits by encouraging you to keep your hands up and react quickly after throwing. It's especially useful for building fluid offensive and defensive sequences. Each strike triggers the bar's return, giving you a chance to practice ducking, blocking, or countering in rhythm. Over time, it helps develop timing, coordination, and the ability to transition smoothly between offense and defense.

Maize Ball: A small, hanging bag often filled with sand or other material, designed to swing unpredictably. Used by legends like Mike Tyson, it's ideal for drilling head movement, slips, and defensive rhythm. The constant motion forces you to react on instinct, improving your ability to evade punches while staying balanced.

Wall Bag: A compact striking surface mounted directly to a wall, used to develop punching technique, accuracy, and power without the swinging movement of a heavy bag. Its fixed position forces you to generate force through proper mechanics rather than relying on bag momentum. Wall bags are great for practicing straight punches, hooks, and uppercuts with consistent impact, making them an excellent tool, especially in small spaces where larger bags won't fit.

Ropes for Slipping Under: A simple but effective setup where a rope is stretched horizontally across the gym at head height. Fighters weave under the rope while throwing punches, developing smooth, efficient head movement in sync with their offense. This drill reinforces proper mechanics, defensive instincts, and builds the kind of rhythm, timing, and endurance needed to operate effectively in mid- to close-range exchanges.

Slip-Sticks: A stick or padded tool that a coach swings at your head, requiring them to slip, weave, and counter. This tool develops fast reactions, defensive awareness, and counterpunching skills by forcing fighters to stay present and adjust to sudden attacks.

Chapter 23
Periodization: Structured Training for Peak Performance

This chapter lays out a complete framework designed to get a fighter to peak condition, but you're not expected to apply everything at once. Think of it as a blueprint. Use what serves you now, and return to the rest as your training evolves. Even world-class fighters build up to this level over time. This is a guide, not a checklist.

Think of periodization like planning a road trip. You have a final destination (your peak performance before a fight), but you can't drive straight there without making stops along the way. Each phase of your training is like a rest stop, where you focus on specific goals to recharge and refuel, so you're ready for the next stretch of your journey.

Without periodization, you risk overtraining, burnout, or hitting a performance plateau. A well-structured plan helps you avoid these issues while improving your overall fitness and ensuring you're ready to perform at your best when it counts.

The High/Low System: Training Efficiently

A simple way to apply periodization on a weekly basis is through the High/Low System. On high days, you push yourself with intense workouts, while low days focus on lighter activities to allow your body to recover.

How the High/Low System Works

High Days: These involve tough boxing sessions, strength training, and conditioning exercises.

Low Days: These are for light activities like cardio, stretching, and mobility exercises to help your body recover and avoid overtraining.

Balancing Intensity and Spacing Workouts

When you're combining different types of training—like sparring, strength work, conditioning, and road work—it's crucial to think about how you space out your workouts. Proper spacing ensures your body has time to recover and perform at its best in every session.

Why Spacing Out Workouts Matters

Optimizes Performance: If you do two intense workouts back-to-back, your second session might suffer due to fatigue. Spacing workouts by several hours or splitting them between morning and evening sessions helps you perform better in both.

Aids Recovery: The more demanding a workout, the more rest your body needs to rebuild and adapt. Sparring, strength training, and intense conditioning all require focused recovery time.

Prevents Overtraining: Structured spacing in your training, especially when alternating between high and low intensity, helps avoid burnout, chronic fatigue, and injury, keeping your body fresh and performance-ready.

Best Practices for Spacing Workouts

Morning and Evening Sessions: If your schedule allows, train twice a day by doing sparring or conditioning in the morning, then follow with strength training or technical drills later in the day.

Minimum Recovery: Aim for at least four to six hours rest in between intense sessions. This will give your body time to refuel and reset, ensuring you're ready to perform.

Listen to Your Body: Always monitor how your body feels between sessions. If you're feeling fatigued, consider adding more time between workouts or moving a session to the next day.

Aerobic and Anaerobic Training

Understanding the balance between aerobic and anaerobic training is crucial to making the High/Low system work. Think of aerobic training as filling up your gas tank with fuel, providing the endurance you need for long rounds. Anaerobic training is like turbocharging your engine, giving you those short, powerful bursts of speed and strength when you need them most.

Aerobic Training

Aerobic training involves activities that you can sustain for longer periods (typically 30 minutes to an hour or more at a steady pace). These workouts rely on oxygen to fuel your muscles and build endurance. Think of it as the engine that keeps you going round after round.

Why You Need Aerobic Training

Builds endurance: Aerobic training improves your cardiovascular health, helping you last longer in the ring.

Aids recovery: By improving blood flow and oxygen delivery, aerobic exercises help you recover faster between exchanges in a fight and maintain output over multiple rounds.

Supports weight management: Aerobic training helps regulate body fat levels, making it easier to stay within your weight class when combined with proper nutrition.

Anaerobic Training

Anaerobic training focuses on short, intense bursts of energy that don't rely on oxygen. This is where you build strength, speed, and explosiveness—like firing up that turbo boost for a powerful sprint or punch.

Why You Need Anaerobic Training

Builds power: Short, intense workouts train your muscles to deliver explosive force.

Increases speed: Anaerobic exercises make you faster and more effective, allowing for quick offensive and defensive movements.

Prepares you for intensity: This training helps you handle high-intensity moments during a fight, like throwing rapid combinations or defending against an onslaught.

By balancing aerobic training on low days and anaerobic training on high days, you ensure a well-rounded training plan that builds both endurance and power.

Peaking for Perfection: Reaching Your Fight Night Pinnacle

In the weeks leading up to a fight, your goal is to "peak": arriving at your absolute best physically and mentally, just before stepping into the ring.

At the highest levels of the game, victory often comes down to who shows up better *that night*. Peaking properly needs to be more than just being in shape, it's about making sure your sharpest, most explosive, and most focused self shows up on fight night. When two well-prepared fighters meet, the one who's dialed in at just the right moment often walks away with the win.

What Does Peaking Look Like?

Maximum Physical Conditioning: You're at your strongest, fastest, and most powerful.

Sharpened Techniques: Your boxing skills are polished and precise.

Mental Focus: You're mentally clear, confident, and ready to execute your game plan.

Optimal Recovery: Your body feels fresh and well-rested, with minimal fatigue.

How Training Camp Helps You Peak

Your training camp is structured to help you build toward your peak gradually. With the right balance of hard work and strategic rest, you'll be ready to perform at your best on fight night.

Building Up: In the early weeks, you gradually increase the intensity, building strength, speed, and endurance.

Strategic Rest: Recovery days allow your body to heal and grow stronger.

Skill Sharpening: As the fight nears, you focus more on technical drills and sparring to perfect your skills.

Mental Preparation: Visualization and game planning ensure you're mentally prepared for the fight.

Tapering Off: In the final week, you reduce intensity, allowing your body to fully recover and dial in for the fight.

Example of an 8-Week Periodization Plan

Here's an example of an 8-week periodization plan leading up to a 10-round professional fight. This section focuses solely on the boxing-specific aspects of periodization, such as sparring, technical drills, and overall fight preparation.

While road work (running) is included here as part of boxing preparation, the Strength & Conditioning (S&C) section on Mesocycles will cover additional conditioning methods, including other forms of cardio, strength work, and power development.

Note for Amateurs: This plan is designed for fighters preparing for professional-level bouts with longer rounds. If you're an amateur, this plan may not be ideal for you, as it's structured around more intense fight preparation. However, you can still benefit from the principles of periodization, especially the High/Low system, which will help you manage your training load and recovery. Adjust the intensity and volume to suit your current level and goals.

Weeks 1-2: General Preparation Phase

Goal: Build a strong aerobic and technical foundation. Sparring is limited to twice per week (Tuesday and Saturday) to avoid early fatigue.

Include longer steady-state runs (3 to 5 miles at a steady pace, staying within Zone 2, can be 30 to 60 minutes depending on individual pace).

Zone 2 refers to a moderate intensity where your heart rate is elevated, but you can still carry on a conversation without feeling out of breath. You're working, but it's sustainable for longer periods, ideal for building the endurance needed for later stages of fight preparation. (Note: You'll often pass through Zone 3 during boxing-specific drills or mitt work, but it's not necessary to target it deliberately in your road work or conditioning.)

The sparring increases by two rounds in week two.

> **Monday (Low):** Technical drills, mitt work, shadowboxing, road work (3 to 4 miles, Zone 2, 30-60 minutes).
>
> **Tuesday (High—Sparring Day):** Sparring (4 rounds → 6 rounds in week two), mitt work.
>
> **Wednesday (Rest):** Rest or Active recovery.
>
> **Thursday (High):** Mitt work, sprint intervals or fartlek run, S&C.

Friday (Low): Technical drills, shadowboxing, road work (three miles, Zone 2, 30-40 minutes).

Saturday (High—Sparring Day): Sparring (4 rounds → 6 rounds in week 1), heavy bag, S&C (after sparring).

Sunday: Full rest day.

Weeks 3-4: Specific Preparation Phase

Goal: Develop boxing-specific endurance and refine techniques and tactics. Sparring increases to 3 times per week (Tuesday, Thursday, Saturday).

Monday (Low): Technical drills, shadowboxing, road work (4 to 5 miles, Zone 2, 40-60 minutes).

Tuesday (High—Sparring Day): Sparring (6 rounds), mitt work, S&C (after sparring).

Wednesday (Low): Road work (3 to 4 miles., Zone 2, 30 minutes).

Thursday (High—Sparring Day): Sparring (6 rounds → 8 rounds in week four), mitt work, S&C (after sparring).

Friday (Rest): Full rest day.

Saturday (High—Sparring Day): Sparring (6 rounds → 8 rounds in week 4), heavy bag, S&C (after sparring).

Sunday (Rest): Full rest day.

Weeks 5-6: Pre-Competition Phase

Goal: Peak power and sport-specific conditioning. Sparring remains at three sessions per week but now reaches 10 rounds to match fight demands. If well-recovered, you may add two additional rounds (up to 12) in week six at your own discretion.

Some elite professionals push beyond this, sparring 12-15+ rounds. However, remember that fight preparation is about sharpening, rather than just grinding. Make sure any extra rounds are purposeful and high-quality, not simply for added volume. If you extend rounds, ensure recovery is prioritized so you enter fight week feeling explosive, not fatigued.

Include sprint intervals (6 to 8 reps of 100m sprints) in Zone 4-5, which are high-intensity sprinting efforts designed to develop power and anaerobic capacity.

Zone 4-5 refers to near-maximal and maximal intensity efforts. In Zone 4, you're working at 80-90% of your max heart rate—breathing is heavy, and sustaining this effort is difficult for long durations. In Zone 5, you're at 90-100% of your max heart rate—this is an all-out sprint effort where talking is impossible, and fatigue sets in quickly. These sprint intervals mimic the anaerobic bursts needed for explosive exchanges in a fight.

> **Monday (Low):** Technical drills, shadowboxing, road work (4-5 miles, Zone 2, 40-60 minutes).

> **Tuesday (High—sparring Day):** Sparring (8 rounds → 10 rounds), mitt work, strength training, sprint intervals (6 to 8 reps of 100m sprints, Zone 4-5).

> **Wednesday (Rest):** Full rest day.

> **Thursday (High—sparring Day):** Sparring (8 → 10 rounds in week 6), mitt work, strength training, sprint intervals (6 to 8 reps of 100m sprints, Zone 4-5).

> **Friday (Low):** Technical drills, shadowboxing, road work (4 miles, Zone 2, 30-50 minutes).

> **Saturday (High—Sparring Day):** Sparring (8 rounds → 10 rounds), light mitt work, S&C.

> **Sunday:** Rest.

Week 7: Tapering & Peaking

Goal: Maintain sharpness while beginning the final taper. Reduce overall volume, but keep high-quality work.

> **Monday (Low):** Technical drills, shadowboxing, road work (3-4 miles, Zone 2, 30-50 min).

Tuesday (High—Sparring Day): Sparring (6 rounds), mitt work, sprint bursts (4 to 6 reps of 50-75m sprints, 90% effort, Zone 4-5).

Wednesday (Rest): Full rest day.

Thursday (High—Sparring Day): Sparring (4 rounds), light mitt work, sprint bursts (4 reps of 50m sprints, 90% effort, Zone 4-5).

Friday (Low): Shadowboxing, footwork drills, road work (3 miles, Zone 2, 30-50 minutes).

Saturday (High—Final Hard Session): Fight-paced mitt work, explosive bag work, short sprint intervals (3 to 4 reps of 50m sprints, 90% effort, Zone 4-5), and final S&C session. Optional light technical sparring (2 to 3 rounds).

Sunday: Rest.

Week 8: Fight Week

Goal: Ensure complete recovery and mental preparation.

Monday: Light technical training, shadowboxing, light bag work, optional light 2 to 3 mile jog.

Tuesday: Rest.

Wednesday: Light shadowboxing, technical drills, light mitt work, optional light 2 to 3 mile jog.

Thursday: Rest.

Friday: Light shadowboxing, visualization and mental preparation.

Saturday: Fight Night.

Sparring Progression

Week	Rounds Per Sparring Session
1	4-6
2	6
3	6-8
4	8
5	8-10
6 (PEAK)	10
7	6, then taper to 4
8 (Fight Week)	Maximum 4 rounds, only light work

Training Intensity and Tapering for Peak Performance

This plan gradually increases the intensity and specificity of your training over the 8 weeks. As fight night approaches, the training volume decreases during the final week. This is called tapering. The goal is to allow your body to fully recover and reach its peak when it matters most.

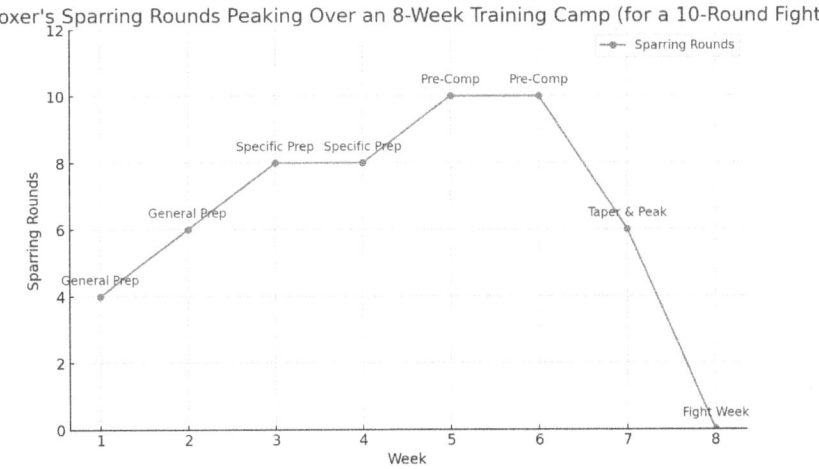

Boxer's Sparring Rounds Peaking Over an 8-Week Training Camp (for a 10-Round Fight)

The High/Low System is used throughout the 8 weeks to manage fatigue and optimize recovery. By alternating between high-intensity sessions and lighter recovery days, you avoid overtraining and stay sharp.

Listening to Your Body

Recovery is just as important as the hard work you put in, and no two fighters are the same. While this plan provides a solid framework, it's important to remember that everyone's body reacts differently to training. This is just an example. Your training plan should be tailored to your individual needs and adjusted as you go.

Remember, take days off as needed. Recovery is key. This isn't cookie cutter. Although you need a team to compete at the highest level, boxing is an individual sport once that bell rings. Everyone is different and you must *listen to your body*. If your body is giving you signals that you need to take a day or two off, do it! Your team (coaches, trainers, and medical staff) can provide invaluable advice, but ultimately, you know your own body best.

Here is a graph showing the progression of sparring rounds during an 8-week training camp for a 10-round fight. The number of sparring rounds increases progressively, peaking in the middle weeks, and then tapers off in the final week to ensure optimal readiness and recovery for fight night. The annotations indicate the different phases of the training camp.

Understanding Reversibility and Its Impact on Boxing Performance

As you prepare for a fight, it's important to grasp how quickly different fitness qualities diminish when they're not consistently worked on. This concept, known as *Reversibility*, helps you keep your body primed for peak performance on fight night. Each fitness attribute, whether it's endurance, strength, or speed, holds on for different lengths of time once developed. That's why timing your training can be a major strategic advantage.

Breaking It Down for Boxing Training

This table gives you a clear idea of how long each physical ability remains effective after you stop training it regularly, and why each one is important for your boxing performance. Here's the breakdown:

Aerobic Endurance (Gas Tank Endurance) is like the engine that keeps you going throughout all rounds. Once you build it up, it typically lasts for about 30 days, give or take 5 days, without much direct training. That means you don't need to focus on it daily once it's established. This is your ability to keep moving and throwing punches for many rounds without getting exhausted. It's what keeps you bouncing on your toes, circling the ring, and jabbing steadily throughout a fight.

Example Exercises: Long-distance running, cycling, or swimming for 30 to 60 minutes at a steady pace. These build stamina to maintain energy over long rounds.

Maximal Strength (Raw Power) gives you the raw force to make your punches land with authority. Like aerobic endurance, it stays with you for around 30 days, plus or minus 5 days, after you stop focusing on it. So, you can shift focus to other areas while still maintaining strength. This is the force behind your punches and clinch control, what helps you land a big shot or move an opponent when needed.

Example Exercises: Heavy lifts like squats, deadlifts, and bench presses with low reps to build raw strength, the foundation behind hard-hitting punches. Olympic lifts like power cleans and snatches also enhance strength and explosiveness, bridging raw power and speed.

Anaerobic Glycolytic Endurance (Fight Pace Endurance) allows you to push through hard combinations without getting gassed too quickly. This quality starts to fade faster, usually after 18 days, plus or minus 4 days, so you need to keep working on it regularly throughout camp. This energy system kicks in during high-intensity bursts, like flurries of punches or the final seconds of a tough round, helping you fight through fatigue when your body can't get enough oxygen.

Example Exercises: Sprint intervals, circuit training with battle ropes and burpees, or intense bag work sessions. This builds the capacity to handle explosive movements and recover quickly between rounds.

Strength Endurance (Sustained Output) ensures your muscles can keep going over long periods. This is key for maintaining power throughout multiple rounds. It begins to diminish after about 15 days, plus or minus 5 days, so refresh it regularly to stay strong over time. This quality supports repeated combinations and clinch work without your punches losing impact in the later rounds.

Example Exercises: Kettlebell swings, high-rep bodyweight squats, or push-up variations. These train your muscles to endure continuous high output during fights.

Maximal Speed (Alactic) (Explosive Speed) fades the quickest, lasting only around 5 days, give or take 3 days. This is why you focus on speed and explosiveness closer to fight night, ensuring you're at your sharpest when it matters. This system supports short bursts of 6–10 seconds, so rest between sets is crucial to avoid fatigue and maintain explosiveness. This is what powers lightning-quick jabs, sudden counters, or fast slips—short bursts of top-end speed.

Example Exercises: Short sprints (20-40 meters), explosive medicine ball throws, or plyometric jump training. These target fast-twitch muscles for rapid, decisive movements like delivering knockout punches or dodging attacks.

How This Fits Into Your Training Program

Understanding Reversibility helps you plan your training smarter. Here's how it fits into your 8-week boxing S&C program:

Weeks 1-2: Focus on building strength endurance and aerobic capacity. Aerobic fitness takes longer to develop but lasts longer once built. Strength endurance is trained early because it helps prevent injuries, improves fatigue resistance, and lays the foundation for heavier strength work in later phases. Developing this endurance now ensures that when you transition to maximal strength and power work, your muscles and connective tissues are prepared to handle increased loads, and you can sustain those outputs across multiple rounds.

Weeks 3-4: Shift focus to building maximal strength. Since strength can be maintained for up to 30 days with reduced frequency, you can then transition into more explosive and anaerobic work while keeping strength gains intact.

Weeks 5-6: Emphasize anaerobic glycolytic endurance and power endurance , the ability to sustain explosive, high-intensity efforts across rounds. These qualities decay faster than strength or aerobic fitness but are crucial for sustaining high-intensity bursts and explosive movements during fight exchanges. Strength endurance may also be included to support volume and muscular stamina.

Weeks 7-8: Maximize speed and explosiveness in the tapering phase. Since speed deteriorates the fastest, this is the perfect time to sharpen explosiveness, fine-tune reaction time, and ensure you're at peak fight-night readiness.

Why This Matters for Your Fight

In boxing, timing is everything, not limited to the ring but in your preparation as well. By knowing how long each fitness quality lasts, you can time your training to peak at the perfect moment. Beyond putting in the work; you're focusing on what will matter most when you step into the ring.

Picture yourself on fight night. Your endurance is ready to carry you through every round, your strength fuels every punch, and your speed keeps you one step ahead. You've trained efficiently, keeping your body primed in all the right areas. There's no wasted effort, no unnecessary fatigue, just a finely tuned machine ready for war.

This approach ensures that when the bell rings, you're not only in good shape, but you're also in the best shape possible, with every key physical quality sharpened and ready to help you dominate. You've maximized your preparation to ensure that you're at your peak when it matters most.

Mesocycles for Boxing S&C: An 8-Week Program

Welcome to your 8-week Strength and Conditioning (S&C) program designed specifically for professional-level boxers getting ready for a fight. While this program is intense and highly structured to meet the demands of a professional bout, it can also serve as a solid framework for advanced amateurs looking to take their training to the next level. That said, remember that your boxing training is the most important part of your preparation. This S&C plan is meant to complement, not replace, your technical boxing work.

This chapter outlines an 8-week S&C program, but mesocycles are more than fight camps. These structured training blocks can be used year-round to develop key physical attributes like endurance, strength, power, and speed. If you're in camp, you can align mesocycles with your boxing periodization, but they don't have to follow the exact same structure.

The previous chapter focused on boxing periodization: how to structure your sparring, roadwork, and technical work to peak for a fight. Now, we'll focus on S&C mesocycles, ensuring your physical attributes are developed in the most effective way possible.

This is an example program designed with high-level professional demands in mind. It's important to tailor the intensity and workload to your individual recovery and fitness levels. Working with a qualified coach or specialist is highly recommended to ensure the program aligns with your needs and is performed correctly. Every fighter is different, so following a plan that works best for your body will help you get the most out of your training while avoiding overtraining or injury.

What's the Difference Between Periodization and Mesocycles?

Periodization is your long-term training strategy: it's like the master plan for the entire road trip. It organizes your training over weeks or months to ensure you're peaking at the right time for fight night.

Mesocycles are the phases within that strategy, like individual stops along the way. Each mesocycle has a specific goal, whether it's building endurance, increasing strength, or sharpening speed.

To make this even clearer:

Term	Think of it like this	Purpose
Periodization	Planning a cross-country road trip.	Organizing your entire training over weeks/months to reach peak performance.
Mesocycles	The stops along the road trip.	Focused training blocks (two to four weeks each) with specific goals (strength, power, endurance, etc.).

By understanding the difference, you'll see how periodization gives you the big picture and mesocycles focus on building specific attributes at the right time.

How Periodization Works with Mesocycles

Periodization ensures your training progresses smoothly, while mesocycles allow you to focus on specific physical and technical adaptations during each phase.

Now that you understand the big-picture approach of periodization, let's break it down further. Your training is divided into mesocycles, each designed to build a specific attribute at the right time.

Understanding Mesocycles

Imagine you're forging a powerful weapon, something sharp and unstoppable. Each mesocycle is a step in this process. First, you heat the metal to make it flexible: that's your strength endurance phase, where you build a base of endurance and aerobic capacity. Then, you hammer that metal into shape, turning it into something solid and unbreakable. This is where you focus on general strength. Next, you sharpen the edges, giving it lethal precision, this is your power endurance phase, where speed and explosiveness take over. Finally, you polish and fine-tune it, making sure it's perfectly balanced and ready to strike with maximum impact. That's your speed and peaking phase, right before fight night.

By the time you've finished this process, you've crafted the ultimate weapon: yourself. Strong, fast, and ready to unleash everything you've built when it counts the most.

For this 8-week program, we'll use four mesocycles:

1. **Strength Endurance and Aerobic Capacity Phase (Weeks 1-2):** Lay down the raw material by building muscular endurance and aerobic capacity to support everything that comes after.

2. **General Strength Phase (Weeks 3-4):** Shape your strength, making it tough and durable to handle the demands of the ring.

3. **Power Endurance Phase (Weeks 5-6):** Sharpen your speed and explosiveness, turning your raw power into precise, fight-ready movements.

4. **Speed and Peaking Phase (Weeks 7-8):** Refine and fine-tune everything, ensuring you're razor-sharp and at your absolute best for fight night.

Strength & Conditioning Frequency in Fight Camp

How often should you do S&C while preparing for a fight? The answer depends on your overall workload, recovery, and physical needs. Here's a breakdown of the most effective training frequencies based on fight camp demands:

Sessions	Best For	Potential Issues
2x per week (Minimal Dose)	Maintenance of strength and power while prioritizing boxing workload.	May not be enough to drive adaptations, but works well for skill-heavy fight camps.
3x per week (Balanced Approach)	Allows a proper balance of strength, power, and conditioning while focusing on boxing.	Needs good recovery management to avoid fatigue interfering with boxing.
4x per week (High Volume Camp)	Fighters who need more S&C development (e.g., those who started camp out of shape).	High risk of overtraining, must be carefully programmed to avoid diminishing boxing performance.

In general, during the early stages of fight camp (weeks 1-4), S&C can be done 3x per week or more, to build or reinforce strength and conditioning. As the fight nears (Weeks 5-8), S&C should taper down to 2x per week to avoid interfering with sharpness and skill work.

8-Week Boxing S&C Program

Mesocycle 1: Strength Endurance and Aerobic Capacity Phase (Weeks 1-2)

Explanation: In this phase, you'll focus on strength endurance exercises and aerobic capacity work, which lays the groundwork for everything else. Like heating metal to make it malleable, you're preparing your body to handle the upcoming intense phases. The high repetitions of strength endurance training will primarily target the slow-twitch muscle fibers responsible for endurance, while also tapping into fast-twitch fibers as fatigue sets in. Meanwhile, aerobic capacity training enhances your cardiovascular system, improving the body's ability to deliver oxygen to your muscles over long periods.

Goal: Develop muscular endurance and aerobic capacity to create a strong base for future phases.

Monday (Moderate): Strength endurance exercises and calisthenics (higher reps with moderate weights: kettlebell swings, medicine ball throws, jump squats, push-ups, bodyweight lunges).

Tuesday (Low): Aerobic capacity training (steady-state cardio like a 30-60-minute jog, bike ride, or swimming).

Wednesday (High): Sprint intervals and conditioning (6 x 100m sprints with 90 seconds rest, followed by battle ropes and burpees).

Thursday (Low): Aerobic capacity training (30-60 minute jog or swim, maintaining a steady pace).

Friday (Moderate): Upper body strength endurance, core work, and calisthenics (plyometric push-ups, medicine ball slams, hanging leg raises, pull-ups, dips).

Saturday (High): High-intensity interval training (HIIT).

Sunday: Rest.

Mesocycle 2: General Strength Phase (Weeks 3-4)

Explanation: Now that your body is prepped, you'll start forging it with general strength training. In this phase, you're hammering that flexible material into something solid and durable, using heavier weights with lower repetitions. This work primarily targets the fast-twitch muscle fibers, which are responsible for strength and short bursts of explosive power. While you continue to maintain your aerobic base, the focus shifts to raw strength, preparing your body to handle intense physical demands.

Goal: Build a strong foundation of strength, reinforcing the endurance base you've built, to support the explosive work ahead.

Monday (Moderate): Full-body strength training (squats, deadlifts, bench press, rows).

Tuesday (Low): Steady state cardio, mobility work (30-60 minute jog, bike ride, or swimming; stretching).

Wednesday (High): Plyometrics and high-intensity cardio (box jumps, burpees, followed by sprints or interval swimming).

Thursday (Low): Steady state cardio, mobility work (30-60 minute swim or elliptical; yoga).

Friday (Moderate): Upper body strength, core work, and calisthenics (pull-ups, dips, planks, Russian twists, push-ups).

Saturday (Low): Recovery activities (light cardio, foam rolling, dynamic stretching).

Sunday: Rest.

Mesocycle 3: Power Endurance Phase (Weeks 5-6)

Explanation: With a solid foundation in place, it's time to sharpen your edges. In this phase, you'll focus on power endurance exercises that blend strength and speed. Movements like power cleans and box jumps take the raw strength you've built and turn it into quick, explosive power. This phase targets both slow-twitch and fast-twitch muscle fibers, ensuring you can sustain explosive movements over long periods. It's about turning your raw power into precise, fight-ready movements.

Goal: Sharpen your power and speed, ensuring your movements are explosive and fight-ready.

Monday (Moderate): Power endurance exercises and calisthenics (power cleans, box jumps, explosive step-ups, push-ups, bodyweight squats).

Tuesday (Low): Light cardio, recovery work (30-45-minute light jog; stretch).

Wednesday (High): Post-Activation Potentiation (PAP) and intense cardio (heavy back squat followed by vertical jumps, bench press followed by explosive push ups, finishing with sprints).

Note: PAP is a training technique that combines a heavy strength movement with an explosive exercise. This method enhances your muscles' power output by priming them with a heavy lift, followed by a fast, explosive movement. It activates your nervous system to produce more force and speed during explosive movements in the ring.

Thursday (Low): Steady state cardio, mobility work (30-45 minutes on a stationary bike; stretching).

Friday (Moderate): Power endurance, core work, and calisthenics (sledgehammer strikes, battle ropes, Turkish get-ups, pull-ups, dips).

Saturday (High): Mixed high-intensity conditioning (sprints followed by circuit training).

Sunday: Rest

Example Circuit Training Routine
(30 seconds work/15 seconds rest for 8 rounds):

- Push-ups
- Bodyweight Squats
- Burpees
- Mountain Climbers
- Plank to Push-up
- Jumping Lunges
- High Knees
- Russian Twists

Instructions: Repeat the circuit for the desired number of rounds, taking a 1- to 2-minute rest between rounds if needed.

Mesocycle 4: Speed and Peaking Phase (Weeks 7-8)

Explanation: In the final phase, you're honing your weapon. To ensure it's sharp, fast, and ready for fight night. The focus here is on speed work and fine-tuning your conditioning. Movements become lighter but more precise, with an emphasis on quickness and agility. You're not building anymore; you're preparing to unleash everything you've worked for. By tapering your workload, you ensure your body is fully recovered and peaked for the fight, allowing you to strike with maximum speed and impact.

Goal: Accentuate your speed, quickness, and agility, ensuring you're in peak condition come fight night.

Week 7: Tapering and Speed Development

Monday (Moderate): Light power training, short sprints, and calisthenics (medicine ball throws, 4 x 20m sprints at 90% effort, push-ups, bodyweight lunges).

Tuesday (Low): Light cardio, mobility work (30-minute light jog, stretching).

Wednesday (Low): Light full-body circuit, core work, and calisthenics (bodyweight exercises, plank variations).

Thursday: Rest.

Friday (Low): Light cardio and dynamic stretching (20-30-minute jump rope; mobility drills).

Saturday (Moderate): Short, high-intensity session with calisthenics (3 rounds of 2-minute high-intensity circuit work, followed by sprints).

Sunday: Rest.

Week 8: Fight Week

Monday (Low): Light mobility work, stretching (joint rotations, light yoga).

Tuesday: Rest.

Wednesday (Low): Very light cardio and dynamic stretching (15-20-minutes of light cardio; dynamic stretching routine).

Thursday: Rest.

Friday (Low): Light activation exercises and stretching. Some fighters may opt for a short shakeout or light pad session on Friday to stay loose, depending on their routine and how their body feels.

Saturday: Rest (Fight Day).

Implementation Guidelines

Progression: Start with lower intensity and volume, gradually increasing through the first three phases. In the final phase (taper), reduce both to allow for recovery.

Individualization: Tailor the exercises and intensity to match your own strengths, weaknesses, and how well you recover.

Integration: This S&C program works best when combined with your boxing training, it shouldn't replace your technical practice.

Monitoring: Pay attention to how your body feels. If you're overly tired, rest and adjust your workouts as needed.

Recovery: Make sure to eat well, stay hydrated, and get plenty of sleep to help your body recover.

Flexibility: While the program is structured, it's important to make adjustments based on how you're feeling.

Cardio Options: Choose the type of cardio that suits you and keeps you engaged. Changing up your routine can prevent boredom and improve your overall conditioning.

Remember: This plan is a starting point. Customize it to fit your specific needs, fitness level, and how your body responds. If something doesn't feel right, take rest days or modify the workouts. Consulting with a coach or specialist is always helpful.

This eight-week mesocycle-based S&C program is designed to help you get in the best shape possible for your fight. By working through the different phases like building endurance, maximizing strength, increasing power, and enhancing speed, you'll reach your peak on fight night.

Chapter 24
The Pulse of Performance: Heart Rate Zones

"Training without a heart rate monitor is like driving without a speedometer." [47]
—Stu Mittleman, endurance master

In boxing, your heart is more than just a muscle; it's your internal motor. Whether you're starting your journey or striving to become a world-class fighter, understanding how to manage your heart rate during training can make the difference between progress and burnout. By tracking your heart rate zones and using tools like heart rate variability (HRV), you can train smarter, recover better, and perform at your best.

The 5 Heart Rate Zones

Your heart rate changes depending on how hard you're working. By training in different heart rate zones, you can target specific fitness goals, from building endurance to increasing power. The table below outlines the key heart rate zones, their percentage of maximum heart rate, and how each zone benefits boxing performance.

---

[47] Mittleman, Stu. *Slow Burn: Burn Fat Faster By Exercising Slower*. HarperCollins, 2001.

Heart Rate Zone	% of Max HR	Boxing Relevance	Benefits
Very Light	**50-60%**	Recovery, warm-up, cool-down.	Helps you recover between rounds by boosting blood flow and reducing muscle soreness. Also great for warming up before intense sessions or cooling down afterward.
Light	**60-70%**	Building endurance, staying in shape.	Builds endurance and improves recovery, helping you stay fresh during long training sessions and between explosive exchanges. It also enhances overall conditioning for sustained effort in the ring.
Mode-rate	**70-80%**	Improving fitness and stamina.	Builds stamina and helps you maintain a steady pace without fading. This zone improves oxygen efficiency, letting you fight longer at a higher work rate before fatigue sets in.
Hard	**80-90%**	Increasing speed and power.	Trains anaerobic endurance and the ability to sustain high-intensity efforts for longer. This zone pushes your limits in maintaining punching power, hand speed, and explosive footwork under fatigue, crucial for sustained offensive bursts and late-round effectiveness.
Very Hard	**90-100%**	Max effort, KO punches, going for the finish.	Max effort zone for explosive bursts, throwing knockout punches, finishing a fight, or fighting through exhaustion. Trains your ability to deliver power at full intensity when it matters most.

Zone 1: 50-60% Max HR- Very Light

Best for: Recovery, warm-up, and cool-down.

Why: This zone boosts blood flow and helps your muscles recover without added stress. You'll use this for light movement before and after intense sessions.

Zone 2: 60-70% Max HR–Light

Best for: Building endurance, burning fat.

Why: Zone 2 is where you build a solid aerobic foundation, improving your stamina and ability to last through long training sessions or fights. It's perfect for steady, moderate activities like jogging or shadowboxing.

How it feels: Breathing is easy, and you can talk in full sentences. Feels like a relaxed jog, steady jump rope, or light bag work. You'll sweat lightly but won't feel fatigued.

Zone 3: 70-80% Max HR—Moderate

Best for: Improving aerobic fitness.

Why: Training in Zone Three increases your body's ability to use oxygen efficiently, helping you maintain a high level of performance over multiple rounds. It's suitable for light sparring or moderate-paced drills that require consistent movement.

How it feels: Breathing is deeper, and you can talk, but only in short sentences. Feels like a steady-paced run, lower intensity footwork drills, or sustained mitt work. You're working, but it's not exhausting.

Zone 4: 80-90% Max HR—Hard

Best for: Enhancing speed, power, and anaerobic capacity.

Why: Zone 4 pushes you into more intense, high-energy movements, such as throwing fast combinations or quick footwork drills. It improves your ability to sustain high-intensity efforts for longer and enhances your capacity to tolerate fatigue in a fight.

How it feels: Breathing is heavy, and conversation is difficult. Feels like intense sparring, repeated short sprints, or throwing rapid punch combinations. You'll feel the burn in your muscles but can sustain it for shorter periods.

Zone 5: 90-100% Max HR – Maximum Effort

Best for: Peak performance, explosive power.

Why: Zone 5 is where you go all out, training for short, maximum-effort bursts—like a knockout punch or a rapid, forceful combination. Training in this zone builds explosive power, needed for high-stakes moments in a fight.

How it feels: Breathing is extremely heavy, and talking is nearly impossible. Feels like an all-out sprint or throwing continuous high-intensity punch combinations in a fight.

Note: While Zone 4-5 is often associated with short bursts, fighters can stay in this state for nearly an entire round during intense sparring or high-paced fights. However, sustaining this effort requires strong conditioning and controlled energy expenditure to avoid early fatigue.

Calculating Your Maximum Heart Rate

Before you can train effectively within each zone, you need to know your Maximum Heart Rate (Max HR). You can estimate it using this formula:

Max HR = 220 - Age

For example, if you're 25 years old:

220 - 25 = 195 BPM

This formula gives you a general idea, though actual max heart rates can vary slightly based on your fitness level and other factors.

Heart Rate Zones During Boxing Training

As you train, your heart rate will fluctuate depending on the intensity of your workout. This is especially true during a boxing session, where you shift from light warm-ups to all-out efforts in short bursts. The chart below illustrates how your heart rate typically moves through different zones during a boxing training session:

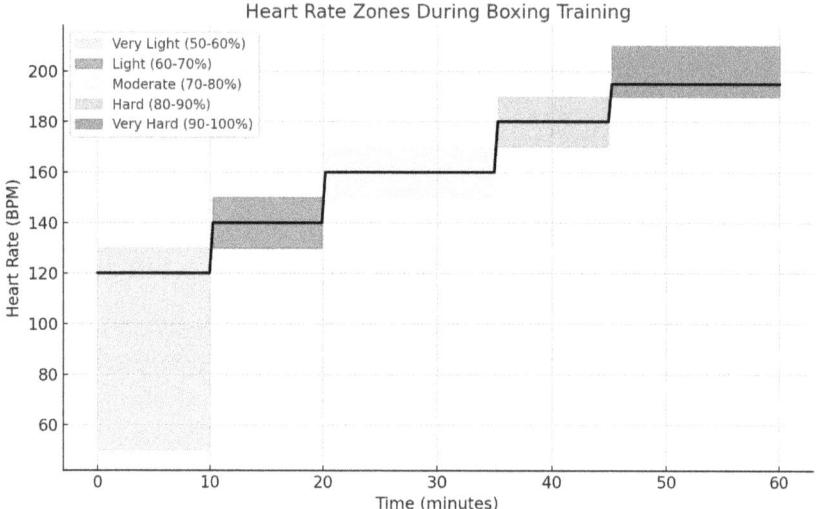

Chart Breakdown:

Very Light (50-60%)—Light Blue: This zone is common during warm-ups and cool-downs, when the body is preparing for or recovering from intense activity. It allows the heart rate to stay low while promoting blood flow.

Light (60-70%)—Green: This zone represents light intensity, such as shadowboxing or light footwork, where you're building aerobic endurance. It's steady but not exhausting.

Moderate (70-80%)—Yellow: As intensity ramps up during steady sparring or moderate-paced bag work, the heart rate increases into this zone. It's where boxers build endurance for lasting multiple rounds.

Hard (80-90%)—Orange: When you're throwing combinations, working the heavy bag, or engaging in intense mitt drills, your heart rate spikes into this zone. This is where anaerobic work begins, building speed and power.

Very Hard (90-100%)—Red: The highest peaks in the chart represent moments of all-out effort, like going for the knockout or finishing a high-intensity interval. This is your maximum effort zone, reserved for short, explosive bursts.

Understanding how your heart rate moves through these zones during training helps you monitor and adjust your intensity for optimal results. There are several ways you can assess your heart rate.

Chest Strap Monitors

Most Accurate: Measures heart rate directly from electrical signals (like an ECG).

Best for High-Intensity Training: Ideal for sparring, conditioning, and detailed tracking.

Less Convenient: Requires wearing a strap around your chest.

> **Examples:** Polar H10, Garmin HRM-Pro.

Wrist-Based Monitors

More Convenient: Built into smartwatches and fitness trackers.

Good for General Training: Suitable for steady-state workouts and everyday use.

Less Accurate During High-Intensity Training: May have lag or inaccuracies during rapid movement.

> **Examples:** Apple Watch, WHOOP, Garmin, Fitbit.

Heart Rate Ranges in a Boxing Match

During a boxing match, heart rate fluctuates significantly depending on the intensity of the action. Here are the typical heart rate ranges a boxer experiences during different phases of a fight:

Resting Between Rounds (100-130 BPM):

- In the 1-minute rest between rounds, a well-conditioned boxer's heart rate should drop into this range.

- Faster heart rate recovery = better conditioning and energy conservation for the next round.

Light to Moderate Effort (140-160 BPM):

- Moving around the ring, feinting, and throwing light jabs keep heart rates in this range.

- This phase allows the boxer to control pace and conserve energy for explosive moments.

High Effort During Intense Exchanges (170-190 BPM):

- Throwing rapid combinations, trading punches, or pressing forward raises heart rates to this range.

- Anaerobic conditioning and lactic acid buildup become major factors here.

Peak Effort (190-200+ BPM):

- During all-out moments, going for a knockout, defending against a flurry, heart rates spike to the max.

- This is Zone 5 ("the red zone"), where boxers are pushed to their absolute limit.

- Common in intense sparring and fights where short, explosive bursts are needed.

Heart Rate Variability (HRV): Train Smarter, Recover Faster

What is HRV?

Heart Rate Variability (HRV) measures the small differences in time between each heartbeat. These variations show how well your body is balancing stress and recovery. A higher HRV means your body is fresh and ready to push harder, while a lower HRV suggests fatigue, stress, or the need for recovery.

How to Track HRV

You need a wearable device like WHOOP, Oura Ring, Apple Watch, Garmin, or Polar H10 to measure HRV. These devices track your HRV overnight or in real time.

Steps to Track HRV Effectively

Use a Device That Tracks HRV: WHOOP, Oura Ring, Polar, and Garmin are popular options.

Measure HRV at the Same Time Every Day: Best done first thing in the morning before training, food, or caffeine.

Find Your Baseline: HRV is unique to you. Track it for one to two **weeks** to see what your normal range is.

Monitor Trends: A one-day drop isn't a big deal, but a consistent downward trend signals overtraining or stress.

How to Use HRV in Training

High HRV (Above Your Baseline)

Your body is recovered and ready for hard training (sparring, intense bag work, sprint intervals).

You can push your limits without excessive fatigue.

Low HRV (Below Your Baseline)

Your body is fatigued, opt for lighter training (technical drills, mobility work, shadowboxing).

Avoid all-out sparring or high-intensity work.

Sudden HRV Drop

If HRV drops significantly from your baseline, you may be overtrained or under-recovered.

Consider an extra rest day to avoid burnout or injury.

Example of HRV Readings Over a Week

Day	HRV (ms)	Resting Heart Rate (BPM)	Training Recommendation
Monday	75 ms (High)	50 bpm (Low)	Hard training
Tuesday	78 ms (High)	48 bpm (Low)	Hard training
Wednesday	45 ms (Low)	62 bpm (High)	Light training
Thursday	50 ms (Low)	60 bpm (High)	Light training
Friday	72 ms (Recovered)	50 bpm (Normal)	Hard training

HRV + Heart Rate Zones = Smarter Training

By combining HRV tracking with heart rate zone training, you can fine-tune your workouts for peak performance. You'll know when to go all out and when to pull back, preventing burnout while maximizing gains.

Key Takeaways for Fighters

HRV tells you when your body is ready for hard training vs. when it needs recovery.

Tracking HRV daily helps prevent overtraining and injury.

HRV trends (not just daily readings) are the best guide for adjusting your workload

Round 5: Physical Development

Chapter 25
Building Your Machine

"When you're talking about fighting, well then, baby, you'd better train every part of your body!" [48]
— Bruce Lee

Boxing is a sport that demands a diverse arsenal of physical attributes in the ring, including strength, speed, endurance, power, balance, and agility. Each of these skills supports the other, helping you become a stronger, more effective fighter.

This guide breaks down the different aspects of conditioning that will help you improve. Whether it's core stability, strength, or explosive power, these elements all work together to shape your overall performance. While the chapters are divided into sections, the reality is that no part of your training stands alone. For example, building strength will also help with endurance, and improving stability will enhance your force.

To keep your body operating at its peak, make sure to loosen up your muscles both before and after your workouts. This helps maintain your speed and fluidity in the ring, ensuring that your body can move freely and respond quickly without stiffness holding you back. It's an important part of staying agile and preventing injuries during training.

How to Use This Guide

This section is designed as a structured roadmap for developing strength, endurance, and power for boxing. However, every fighter is different. Depending on where you're at in your training, you can jump in at any stage or mix and match workouts to fit your needs. This is a long-term development model, it's not a periodization plan for fight camp.

---

[48] Lee, Bruce. *Bruce Lee: The Art of Expressing the Human Body.* Edited by John Little, Tuttle Publishing, 1998.

If you're in a training phase focused on building attributes (off-season or between fights), follow this roadmap to strengthen each layer progressively. However, if you're in fight camp, you should refer to the Mesocycles section within the Periodization chapter for how to structure S&C for your fight preparation while keeping skill work (boxing training) the priority. That section also covers something called "reversibility", or how fast different physical qualities fade if you stop training them—which you might want to check out to better understand how to maintain and maximize your gains.

Both this structured progression and fight camp periodization work together, but they serve different purposes. Think of this section as a blueprint for overall athletic development, while mesocycles fine-tune those attributes at the right time in fight camp.

Think of this guide as a starting framework, a base of information that can be shaped with the help of a coach or tailored on your own to suit your unique development path.

The Training Progression

While you can tailor the workouts to your needs, this is the ideal progression roadmap for building a complete fighter.

Although each phase has a primary focus, no fighter works on just one thing at a time. It's about shifting focus based on what you need most. Use this guide to help structure your training without thinking of each part as a separate stage.

If you're starting fresh, following this order will give you the best results by layering key attributes in the right order. If you're more experienced, you can focus on areas where you need the most improvement while keeping the rest in balance. Think of this as a structured plan, but not a strict rulebook.

You can also incorporate circuit-style training that blends explosiveness, strength, and endurance into continuous workouts. Although circuits aren't part of the structured progression, they're great for maintaining power and conditioning during camp or between fights, especially for amateurs who need to build overall fitness quickly.

Training Roadmap

1. **Core Stability:** The base of all movement, preventing energy leaks and improving balance.

2. **Calisthenics & Light Weights:** Developing endurance, muscular conditioning, and functional strength.

3. **Strength Training:** Building raw strength to hit harder and stay physically dominant.

4. **Olympic Lifts**: Training speed-strength and power expression in controlled movement patterns.

5. **Overcoming Isometrics:** Maximizing force output and muscle activation.

6. **Plyometrics & Functional Power:** Translating strength into explosiveness and endurance.

Conditioning & Endurance: The Other Side of the Equation

While the roadmap focuses on developing strength, speed, and explosiveness, none of it matters without endurance. Cardio ensures you can apply those attributes for as long as the fight lasts.

Continue in "Round 6" (page 292) for the following:

- **Cardiovascular Training for Boxing:** The role of cardio in fight endurance.

- **Running & Roadwork: Building Boxing Stamina:** Classic roadwork, sprint work, and fighter examples.

- **Aquatic Training: Unlocking Superhuman Stamina:** Swimming for endurance, breath control, CO_2 tolerance, and recovery.

- **Cycling & Airdyne Training: Strengthening Leg Stamina:** Supplementary low-impact cardio for endurance.

You don't need strength training to become a great fighter. Plenty of legendary champions dominated the ring without ever touching a barbell, relying instead on cardio, bodyweight work, and relentless fight-specific training. At the same time, many other greats fully embraced strength training and used it to take their power, durability, and performance to the next level. It depends on the kind of fighter you want to become, and how your body responds. That said, no matter which path you follow, I strongly recommend stretching before and after every session to keep your body loose, elastic, and ready to perform, especially if strength work is part of your plan.

That said, when you look at the history of champions, the contrast in approach becomes even clearer. Some of boxing's greatest champions have taken very different approaches when it comes to strength and conditioning. Fighters like Muhammad Ali, Sugar Ray Leonard, and Pernell Whitaker built their dominance without relying on weight training, focusing instead on cardio, calisthenics, and relentless boxing-specific work. On the other hand, fighters like Evander Holyfield, who began using Olympic lifts and a structured S&C program even as a cruiserweight, developed physicality that carried him through heavyweight wars. Artur Beterbiev is a modern example of raw, functional strength. His knockout power comes from serious compound lifting and explosive work. Meanwhile, Terence Crawford blends strength training with mobility and functional drills to stay balanced, strong, and sharp across weight classes.

There's no single blueprint. Greatness has been achieved with, and without, weights. Your job is to find what fits *you* best.

Strength and conditioning (S&C) sessions should generally be done 2-3 times a week. During the off-season, aim for 3 sessions per week to build strength and endurance. If your focus during this period is purely on enhancing athletic ability, you can increase these sessions to 4 or 5 times a week to maximize gains.

Many elite fighters have instinctively followed this same structure, building their physical base before the intensity of fight camp.

Oscar De La Hoya, for example, often did his hardest strength training during the general preparation phase. Once camp began, he dramatically reduced strength work and focused almost entirely on sparring, boxing drills, and fight-specific conditioning.

His goal was to enter camp already physically equipped, so he could devote all his energy to sharpening timing, movement, and ring readiness without added fatigue.

This mirrors the structure laid out here: build the base early, then refine and peak as the fight approaches.

At the same time, aerobic work should remain a consistent part of your training, helping you build the stamina needed for sustained performance in the ring.

Off-Season:

- Long-distance running or steady-state cardio: 2-3 times per week.
- Sprint or interval work: 2-3 times per week.
- Optional: Swimming or cycling for low-impact endurance.

Fight Camp (Closer to a Fight):

- Reduce strength training to 2 sessions per week to maintain power without overtraining.
- Running (long & short intervals): 4–5 times per week.
- Additional cardio (swimming, cycling): 1-2 times per week for recovery and endurance maintenance.

As fight night approaches, your focus should shift from heavy strength work to maintaining endurance, speed, and explosiveness, while minimizing fatigue. Keeping cardio levels on point ensures you enter the ring with the gas tank to go the distance.

The goal is not limited to training hard, it's to train smart. When you understand how each part of your training supports the others, you can design a routine that hits all the right areas, whether you're zeroing in on a weakness or blending methods into a complete system.

In the end, it's about developing the complete package: lasting through tough rounds, delivering power with every punch, and moving with speed and control under fire. This guide will help you build all of that. Making you a more durable, explosive, and dangerous fighter.

Developing the Ultimate Fighter: Strength, Endurance, and Explosive Power

Becoming a physically dominant fighter isn't about excelling in just one attribute. It's about developing strength, endurance, power, balance, and durability into a fully integrated system. Some fighters make the mistake of jumping straight to heavy lifting or plyometrics without first building a solid foundation. True fight performance is a layered process, one that merges multiple elements and evolves over time. While certain methods naturally build on others, your training should be adapted based on your individual needs.

Below is a breakdown of how each training method contributes to your overall physical development and how they can be structured for optimal results. By understanding how these elements fit together, you'll be able to make clear decisions about where to focus your training, ensuring that all aspects of your athleticism are built for peak performance inside the ring.

How Each Training Method Contributes to Power Development

Core Stability → The Foundation for Strength & Power

What it does: Strengthens deep core muscles, improving balance, posture, and energy transfer.

Why it's important: A strong core prevents energy leaks, allowing you to generate force from the ground up.

Limitation: Core stability alone doesn't build strength or explosiveness. It supports them.

Calisthenics & Light Weights → Builds Muscular Endurance & Functional Strength

What it does: Develops high-rep muscular endurance while reinforcing joint stability and body control.

Why it's important: Strengthens key muscle groups without excessive fatigue, helping boxers maintain output across long fights.

Limitation: Doesn't develop maximum force. That comes through heavier strength training.

Strength Training → Builds Maximal Force Production

What it does: Develops raw strength through compound lifts like squats, deadlifts, and presses.

Why it's important: Gives boxers the strength base needed for power and control in exchanges. More strength means the ability to generate higher levels of force with each movement, making punches, clinches, and footwork more powerful.

Limitation: Lifting heavy alone doesn't train explosive movement. It builds force potential, which must be converted into speed and power through later phases.

Olympic Lifts → Develops Strength + Speed, But in Controlled Conditions

What it does: Trains explosive movement in set patterns (e.g., snatches, cleans, jerks).

Why it's important: Helps you apply force quickly, building the ability to move heavy loads fast, a key to explosive punching. At the same time, it develops control and stability, so you don't sacrifice accuracy or balance when delivering that power.

Limitation: Movement is still structured. It doesn't replicate the reactive, unpredictable demands of a real fight.

Overcoming Isometrics → Teaches Maximum Force Output Instantly

What it does: Trains your body to generate max tension instantly by pushing/pulling against immovable resistance.

Why it's important: Primes the nervous system for powerful strikes. Force applied on demand.

Limitation: No movement. Needs to be paired with explosive, dynamic work.

Plyometrics & Functional Training → Converts Strength into Real-Time Explosiveness & Reactivity

What it does: Trains fast, elastic movement in unpredictable, fight-specific ways (jumps, rapid punches, quick lunges, explosive footwork).

Why it's important: This is the final step in the progression. It teaches your body to apply force explosively, repeatedly, and under fatigue.

Key differentiator: Plyometrics develop true speed and reactivity; functional training builds rotational power and explosive endurance that carries into later rounds.

Many fighters also include explosive conditioning circuits during camp, not as part of structured periodization, but as a tool to build endurance under fatigue.

How to Use This Training Progression

This is not a rigid, one-size-fits-all system, but rather a structured roadmap that you can adapt based on where you are in your training. If you have weak core stability, start there before moving into more advanced strength work. If your strength is solid but your explosiveness is lacking, it's time to focus on plyometrics.

Follow the flow, and you'll build not only strength but also the ability to unleash it at will, turning you into a physically dangerous combat athlete.

Now, we begin with the foundation: Core Stability.

Chapter 26
Core Stability: The Secret to Athleticism

The name says it all. The core is a crucial component of movement in boxing. Every punch, slip, and pivot engages the core, but it's beyond strength; it's about stability. A strong, stable core allows for better control, efficient power transfer, and balance in dynamic movements. This chapter will show you how to build core stability and power with targeted exercises.

Core Strength: The Engine of Boxing Performance

Your core is more than just your abs. It includes your lower back, hips, and pelvis, all working together to stabilize your movements and transfer energy from your legs to your upper body. This stability helps you throw stronger punches, maintain balance during footwork, and absorb impact from body shots. While the hips and legs help generate the power, a stable core ensures that energy is transferred efficiently without loss due to poor form.

Key Benefits of Core Stability

Better Balance: A stable core keeps you in control during fast, unpredictable movements, making it easier to dodge punches and stay light on your feet.

Efficient Power Transfer: Core stability ensures that the power generated in your legs and hips travels through your body into your punches with minimal energy loss.

Absorbing Body Shots: A strong core braces your midsection, allowing you to better withstand body shots, reducing their impact and keeping you on your feet.

Injury Prevention: A stable core supports your spine and lower back, reducing the risk of injury from overextension or awkward movements in the ring.

Bruce Lee: The Paragon of Stability

Martial arts legend. Bruce Lee's agility, speed, and striking power were a direct result of his tremendous core stability, which is something every fighter benefits from in the ring. His ability to stay grounded and in control allowed him to generate force while remaining elusive.

One of his most impressive demonstrations of core strength was the Dragon Flag, a movement that required complete control over his body. Lying on a bench, gripping the edge behind his head, he would lift his entire body into the air in a straight line, using only his core strength.

This translated directly into his speed and strength in combat. His ability to stay balanced and centered shows just how important core stability is for any fighter.

Example Core Exercises for Boxing

To build a strong, stable core, these exercises target the muscles you rely on in the ring. Start with the suggested benchmarks and progress over time as your endurance and strength improve.

- **Planks and Variations:** Build core strength and endurance. Side planks also improve oblique strength, helping generate torque for powerful hooks and uppercuts.

How to do it: Hold a plank on your forearms, keeping your body straight and abs tight. For side planks, shift to one arm, position your torso perpendicular to the floor, and hold your body in a straight line. Aim to hold a front plank for 1–2 minutes and side planks for 30–60 seconds per side. Over time, you can build up to adding a weighted plate on your back to further challenge your core and enhance your overall physical performance.

- **Ab Wheel Rollouts:** Strengthen your entire core and lower back, helping you stay balanced while throwing powerful punches.

How to do it: Kneel and roll the ab wheel forward, keeping your body straight, then roll back with control. Start with 6–8 reps per set, focusing on control. Increase volume as strength improves. As your core gets stronger, you can gradually add more sets and reps, or extend the range of motion to challenge your stability even further.

- **Russian Twists:** Strengthen the rotational muscles, key for generating force in punches like crosses and hooks.

How to do it: Sit slightly reclined, then twist your torso side to side while holding a weight. Focus on core control to keep your upper body stable. Perform 20–30 total reps (10–15 per side) with a medicine ball or dumbbell. As you progress, you can increase the weight or speed to improve power and rotational endurance under fatigue.

- **Leg Raises:** Strengthen the lower abs, crucial for staying stable when slipping punches or receiving body shots.

How to do it: Lie on your back with legs extended. Lift your legs to 90 degrees, then lower them slowly, keeping your core tight. Aim for 10–15 controlled reps. As your strength improves, you can add ankle weights to increase the difficulty and further develop lower abdominal control and stability.

- **Turkish Get-Ups:** Develop total-body coordination and unilateral strength, forcing your core to work through multiple planes of motion. This translates to better posture and fluid transitions when throwing combinations or changing levels.

How to do it: Start lying down with a kettlebell in one hand. Slowly rise to standing while keeping the kettlebell overhead. Lower back with control. Begin with 3–5 reps per side using a light-to-moderate weight. As you improve, you can gradually increase the weight or slow down each phase of the movement to build even greater control and full-body stability.

- **Supermans**: Strengthen your lower back and glutes, which support your core and improve stability, especially when defending against body shots. A strong posterior chain also helps maintain punching form and keeps your posture from breaking down in later rounds.

How to do it: Lie face down on the floor with arms extended forward. Lift both arms and legs off the ground simultaneously, squeezing your lower back and glutes. Hold briefly, then lower with control. Aim for 10–15 reps, holding the top position for 2–3 seconds each time. As you get stronger, you can increase the hold time or add light ankle and wrist weights to make the movement more challenging.

Sample Core Circuit:

Perform the following exercises back-to-back with minimal rest. Complete 3–4 rounds, resting 60–90 seconds between rounds.

1. **Front Plank – 60 seconds**
   (Engage your entire core while maintaining posture and breathing under tension.)
2. **Russian Twists – 20 reps total (10 per side)**
   (Use a light-to-moderate weight. Focus on control and full rotation.)
3. **Leg Raises – 12–15 reps**
   (Keep your lower back pressed into the floor and control the lowering phase.)

The Science Behind Core Stability Training

Research shows that core stability improves coordination, increases muscle activation, and boosts athletic performance. A stable core helps you move faster, maintain better balance, and avoid injuries—key advantages for any boxer.[49]

---

[49] Ahmed, et al. "Core Stability and Athletic Performance: A Systematic Review." Journal of Sports Sciences, 2021.

Key Findings

Neuromuscular Control: A strong, stable core sharpens the connection between your brain and muscles, improving reaction time and movement efficiency. In the ring, this means slipping punches with better control, firing counters without losing balance, and recovering quickly from off-angle positions.

Increased Muscle Activation: Core stability training forces multiple muscle groups to work together, strengthening the deep stabilizers that keep your movements crisp and controlled. Over time, this leads to greater endurance, stronger punches, and the ability to maintain explosive movement even in later rounds.

Performance Gains: Fighters with superior core stability move with more speed, power, and balance. A weak core leads to wasted energy and sloppy movement, while a strong one lets you transfer force seamlessly—whether you're throwing a punch, pivoting, or absorbing a shot to the body.

Core Stability for Boxing Success

Building core strength and stability is the foundation of everything you do in the ring. Whether you're throwing punches, dodging an opponent, or absorbing punches, a stable core keeps you in control. These exercises will give you the balance, control, and power needed to excel as a boxer. In the next chapter, we'll build on this foundation by exploring calisthenics, a key tool for combat fitness.

Chapter 27
Calisthenics & Light Weights: Building Endurance and Muscular Conditioning

For decades, calisthenics have been an important part of boxing training because they build the endurance and muscular conditioning boxers need. Whether you're using your own bodyweight or incorporating light weights, these exercises are highly effective at helping you maintain power and speed, round after round.

Reminder: While calisthenics and high-rep training improve muscular endurance, true punch endurance comes from boxing-specific training under fatigue, punching when your arms are tired and maintaining output deep into a fight. Think of these exercises as an additional layer of conditioning, not a replacement for actual fight work.

Why Calisthenics Matter

Endurance: Boxing is a series of repeated movements—punches, footwork, defense. Which all require constant energy. Calisthenics build muscular endurance so you stay sharp, even late in the fight.

Muscular Conditioning: Bodyweight exercises strengthen your muscles to perform effectively even as fatigue sets in, ensuring your punches remain impactful throughout the match.

Functional Strength: Calisthenics work multiple muscle groups at once, developing strength that directly improves your in-ring performance.

Core Strength: As mentioned in the previous chapter, a strong core is essential for generating power, maintaining balance, and absorbing punches. Many calisthenics movements naturally engage the core, helping to develop the stability and strength needed to transfer force efficiently through punches and footwork.

Example Calisthenics Exercises for Boxers

Push-Ups

Benefits: Strengthens the chest, shoulders, and triceps, reinforcing punching endurance and sustained strength. Push-ups help maintain punch volume, pushing strength for inside fighting, and guard endurance throughout each round.

How to Do It: Start in plank position with hands shoulder-width apart. Lower your body until your chest almost touches the ground. Engage your core and keep your body straight. Press back up. For added difficulty, try clap push-ups to build explosiveness.

Variation Tip: Adjust your hand placement to target different angles of the chest and triceps. A wider grip emphasizes the chest more, for hooks and overhands, while a narrow (diamond) grip places more focus on the triceps, reinforcing the endurance needed for straight punches like the jab and cross, where tricep extension is key.

Pull-Ups

Benefits: Strengthens the upper back, biceps, and forearms, improving punch recovery, clinch strength, and maintaining a strong defensive guard. A strong back helps keep the hands up, resist fatigue in long exchanges, and stay defensively sound deep into the fight.

How to Do It: Grab a pull-up bar with your palms facing away. Keep your core tight to prevent swinging and ensure full-body stability. Pull yourself up until your chin clears the bar, then lower yourself with control. The more reps you do, the stronger your grip and upper body become.

Variation Tip: Changing your grip can shift emphasis on different muscle groups. A wide grip mainly targets the lats, helping shoulder stability and punch recovery, while a neutral or underhand grip (chin-up) works the biceps and forearms more, improving inside fighting control and uppercut strength by strengthening the pulling motion needed to drive the punch upward with power.

Dips

Benefits: Strengthens the triceps, chest, and shoulders, increasing punch endurance, short-range power, and clinch control. Dips improve the pressing strength needed for framing, pushing off, and delivering compact, powerful punches like uppercuts and hooks in close range.

How to Do It: Use parallel bars or a sturdy surface, supporting your torso with straight arms. Lower your body by bending your elbows, keeping them close to your sides. Engage your core to keep your body steady and prevent excessive forward lean. Press back up. To make it harder, add weight or slow down each rep.

Variation Tip: Leaning slightly forward will engage the chest more, while keeping a vertical torso focuses more on the triceps, making it a great exercise for punch endurance.

Air Squats

Benefits: Strengthens leg endurance and resilience, keeping your quads, hamstrings, and glutes powerful and responsive for smooth footwork and balance in the ring. A strong lower body enhances explosive movement, stance control, and weight transfer for punching power.

How to Do It: Stand with feet shoulder-width apart. Lower yourself like you're sitting in a chair, keeping your chest up and knees over your toes. Brace your core to stabilize your spine and prevent collapsing forward. Push through your heels to stand back up.

Variation Tip: A narrow stance places more emphasis on the quads, while a wider stance shifts focus to the glutes and inner thighs. Using different stances helps strengthen various movement patterns used in boxing footwork.

Incorporating Light Weights for Additional Conditioning

While calisthenics are highly effective, you can further enhance muscular endurance by using light weights or machines, either separately or alongside your bodyweight exercises. For example, exercises like the dumbbell chest press or leg press with higher repetitions (15+) can push your muscles beyond the bodyweight-only threshold, allowing you to challenge your endurance even more. This method also encourages pushing through "the burn" —the point where muscles are fatigued but need to keep performing—conditioning them to handle the demands of an entire match.

Sample Calisthenics Routine for Endurance

This high-rep routine builds the stamina and muscle conditioning needed to stay sharp and powerful during every phase of the fight:

- **Push-Ups**: 4 sets of 15-20 reps.
- **Pull-Ups**: 4 sets to failure (as many reps as possible).
- **Dips**: 4 sets of 10-15 reps.
- **Air Squats**: 4 sets of 20-30 reps.
- **Optional**: Incorporate light dumbbell or machine exercises, such as dumbbell bench presses or leg presses, for 3 sets of 15-20 reps.

As you get stronger, try harder variations like explosive push-ups or pistol squats (single-leg squats) to further test your endurance.

Safety Tip: Focus on proper form. Maintaining core engagement throughout all movements will improve stability and prevent unnecessary strain on your lower back. Keeping good shoulder alignment will help you avoid injury. Always prioritize control and technique—slow, controlled movements are more effective than fast, sloppy ones.

Key Takeaways

Muscle Endurance: Calisthenics and high-rep weight exercises help you build the endurance needed for sustained effort in a fight.

Core Strength: These exercises naturally engage your core, improving your ability to generate force and stay balanced under fire.

Functional Strength: Each exercise works multiple muscle groups, improving your overall boxing performance.

Scalability: You can increase the difficulty of these exercises as you grow stronger and more conditioned, making them more challenging to keep improving.

Calisthenics and high-rep training build muscular endurance and conditioning, keeping you strong over multiple rounds. But endurance alone won't make your punches devastating. Pure Strength is what turns a well-conditioned fighter into a powerhouse. The stronger you are, the more force you can generate, whether it's for punching, absorbing shots, or bullying your opponent by physically imposing yourself in exchanges and controlling the fight. In the next chapter, we'll break down the foundation of raw strength and how to develop the kind of power that makes opponents think twice before stepping into range.

Chapter 28
Ring Predator: Building Savage Strength

To dominate in the ring, you need raw power, and that starts with building serious strength. Strength training is more than lifting heavy weights. It's about maximizing your body's ability to generate force. Boxing requires full-body strength, from your legs to your core to your upper body.

Research shows that only around 24% of punch power comes from the arms, while the trunk and legs contribute roughly 76%. By training your legs, core, and upper body with compound movements, you build the foundation for powerful punches that can overwhelm opponents.

Safety Tips: Before you start lifting, focus on form and control to avoid injury. Lifting heavy with poor technique can lead to serious setbacks. Always prioritize posture and alignment. Warm up properly, start with manageable weights, and progress gradually as your strength builds. Focus on proper breathing, core engagement, and controlled movement throughout every rep.

Strength Training: The Foundation of Power

Maximal strength is built by lifting heavy weights for low repetitions (typically 3-6 reps per set). Lifting in the 1–2 rep range can also build maximum strength and test absolute limits, but it comes with higher risk. For fighters, the 3–6 rep range hits the sweet spot, allowing you to build serious strength while staying sharp, safe, and well-conditioned.

This range targets fast-twitch muscle fibers, which are responsible for explosive movements. Exercises like squats, deadlifts, military presses, and bench presses are great because they engage multiple muscle groups, preparing your body to generate maximum force.

These exercises can be performed with barbells or dumbbells. Barbells allow for heavier loads, promoting maximal strength and power development, while dumbbells increase range of motion, improve balance, and engage stabilizer muscles. This adds variety to your routine and helps build functional strength, which is key for boxing.

Strength also gives you an edge in physical exchanges, making it harder for opponents to push you around. It also helps your body absorb damage and stay resilient during fatigue-heavy rounds. Many top fighters lift year-round for this very reason, not only for power output, but to maintain a durable frame that holds up under pressure.

Compound Lifts for Boxers

Squats

Benefits: Builds leg power and stability, crucial for generating force from the ground up. Strong legs help you stay balanced and drive through punches during tough exchanges.

How to Do It: Stand with feet shoulder-width apart, chest up, and back straight. Lower your body until your thighs are parallel to the ground, then push through your heels to stand up.

Deadlifts

Benefits: Strengthens the entire body, especially the core and lower back, which are essential for balance and power in your punches.

How to Do It: For the barbell deadlift, stand with feet hip-width apart, grip the bar with hands just outside your knees, keep your back straight, and lift the bar by driving through your legs while engaging your core. If using a trap bar (hex bar), step inside, grip the handles at your sides, and lift while maintaining a neutral spine. This variation reduces lower back strain and allows for a more upright posture, making it great for fighters focused on power and injury prevention.

Military Press

Benefits: Focuses on upper body strength, particularly the shoulders and arms, which are key for delivering strong punches and maintaining your guard.

How to Do It: Stand with feet shoulder-width apart, grip the barbell at shoulder height, and press it overhead. Lower the bar back down with control.

Bench Press

Benefits: Strengthens the chest, shoulders, and triceps, contributing to stronger jabs and crosses. It also improves pushing power for clinches or creating space against your opponent.

How to Do It: Lie on a flat bench, grip the barbell with hands slightly wider than shoulder-width, lower it to your chest, and press it back up while keeping your back flat and feet grounded.

Example Strength Training Routine

- **Squats**: 3 sets of 3-6 reps.
- **Deadlifts**: 3 sets of 3-6 reps.
- **Bench Press**: 3 sets of 3-6 reps.
- **Military Press**: 3 sets of 3-6 reps.

This routine builds a strong base, enhancing your ability to generate force while improving resistance to fatigue.

How Heavy Should You Lift?

When training for strength, choose a weight that feels challenging by the 3rd or 4th rep, but still allows you to complete the set with good form. If you feel like you might fail by the 5th or 6th rep, you're in the right zone. You should finish feeling like you could maybe squeeze out one more, but not two. This keeps you training heavy enough to build maximal strength without sacrificing technique or increasing injury risk.

Will I Gain Weight from Lifting Heavy?

Many boxers worry that lifting heavy weights will add too much muscle and cause them to move up a weight class. However, strength training primarily builds force production and neural efficiency, not bulk. Lifting heavy with low reps (typically 3–5) trains the nervous system to recruit more muscle fibers, increasing strength without significantly increasing size. True hypertrophy (muscle growth) comes from moderate weights and higher reps (typically 8–12 per set).

Boxers also do high amounts of roadwork and conditioning, which, along with clean nutrition, helps regulate body composition and keep weight under control. That said, if you're consistently in a caloric surplus—especially alongside a heavy strength and conditioning workload—some weight gain is still possible. The intense cardio and high-energy demands of a fighter's training naturally burn calories and make excess muscle gain unlikely unless you're actively trying to bulk up.

Stick to strength-based training to build the force foundation for explosiveness, without gaining unnecessary mass or compromising your weight class.

The Role of Strength in Boxing

Strength training gives you the power to control the fight and deliver knockout punches. Whether you're overpowering your opponent or defending against aggressive attacks, a strong foundation ensures you can handle the physical demands of boxing. This training builds force and conditions your muscles to stay strong and durable.

Building raw strength is the base of power, but strength alone won't make you a knockout artist. It must be applied *quickly*, because in boxing, the fastest punch is often the most effective. The next step is learning to convert strength into speed and real-time explosiveness. In the next section, we'll break down Olympic lifts and how they train your body to generate force rapidly, giving you faster, more powerful punches and quicker reactions in the ring.

Olympic Lifts: Where Strength Meets Speed

Once you've built a solid strength base, the next step is converting that strength into dynamic power. Olympic lifts, like power cleans, snatches, and clean and jerks, combine strength with speed, training your body to generate force rapidly. These lifts create fast-twitch, powerful punches and quick reactions in the ring. Other lifts, like the dumbbell push press, also develop rapid-fire strength, boosting your boxing abilities.

If you're unable to perform these barbell exercises or don't have access to barbells, any of these movements can be modified using dumbbells or kettlebells for similar power output benefits.

Attention!

Olympic lifts are highly technical and require proper form to avoid injury. Start light and focus on mastering technique before increasing weight. Lifting heavy with poor mechanics can lead to serious strain, so always prioritize form over load.

- Begin with manageable weights and gradually increase as your technique improves.
- Smooth, controlled movement matters more than the amount of weight lifted.
- If you're lifting heavier loads, consider using a weightlifting belt for lower-back support, especially during clean and jerks or snatches.

If you're unable to perform barbell-based Olympic lifts, you can modify them using dumbbells or kettlebells while maintaining the same explosive intent.

For those looking for a lighter option that still develops quick-strike power, plyometric exercises can be a great alternative. Plyometrics provide similar benefits for speed and reactive power without requiring heavy weights, and will be covered in a later chapter.

Power Cleans

Benefits: Builds explosive power in the legs, hips, and shoulders, directly improving the speed and strength of your punches.

How to Do It: Start with the barbell on the floor, pull it up explosively while keeping the bar close to your body, driving through your hips. Shrug your shoulders and catch the bar at your chest in a slight squat. Stand tall to complete the lift.

Tip: Focus on a strong hip drive and keep your core tight for stability.

Snatches

Benefits: Focuses on speed and full-body explosiveness, helping you generate force quickly, essential for offensive moves in the ring.

How to Do It: Start with the barbell on the floor, pull it up quickly, extending through your hips and shrugging your shoulders, then catch it overhead with arms extended. Drop into a squat before standing up to complete the lift.

Tip: This is a highly technical lift, start light, focus on smooth movement, and keep the bar path close to your body.

Clean and Jerks

Benefits: Develops full-body explosive strength, combining leg power with upper-body force to generate powerful punches and maintain control during close exchanges.

How to Do It: Start with the barbell or on the floor. Perform a clean by pulling the bar to your chest with a strong hip drive. As the bar reaches your shoulders, drop into a front squat to catch it on your chest, then drive back up to standing. From there, dip your knees slightly and explosively drive the bar overhead Use a split stance for stability, then step your feet back together to stand tall and finish the lift.

Tip: Keep your core braced when catching the bar, and focus on stability during the split jerk.

Dumbbell Push Press

Benefits: Develops shoulder, tricep, and core strength while enhancing speed and power, perfect for generating quick-twitch punching power.

How to Do It: Hold a dumbbell in each hand at shoulder height. Dip slightly with your knees, then explosively drive the dumbbells overhead by pushing through your legs and shoulders. Lower with control.

Tip: Use your legs to initiate the movement and ensure a controlled, stable descent.

Olympic Lifts Routine

- **Power Cleans:** 4 sets of 5 reps.
- **Snatches:** 3 sets of 5 reps.
- **Clean and Jerks:** 3 sets of 4-6 reps
- **Dumbbell Push Press:** 4 sets of 6 reps

Perform these lifts at the start of your workout when your energy is high and your focus is sharp. Olympic lifts are all about generating maximum force with each rep, so keep the reps lower to maintain form and snap . Take 2-3 minutes of rest between sets to allow for full recovery and ensure you're performing each set with maximum power.

As you progress, gradually increase the weight to continue building power, but always prioritize proper technique over heavy loads, especially for technical lifts like snatches and clean and jerks.

Key Tip: Start light and perfect your form before increasing the weight. This will help prevent injuries and ensure you're getting the most out of these high-impact lifts.

Rapid power is necessary for delivering fast, devastating punches, but power is only useful if your body can apply it instantly. Strength and speed must be linked together for maximum impact. Overcoming isometrics bridge the gap between raw strength and rapid force production by training your muscles to generate peak force immediately. This method conditions your nervous system to fire with maximal intent from the first millisecond, helping you hit harder and react faster in the ring. In the next chapter, we'll break down how isometrics can take your strength and explosiveness to the next level, making you a more powerful and reactive fighter.

Chapter 29
Overcoming Isometrics: The Force Multiplier

Imagine being able to generate unstoppable force on command. That's what overcoming isometrics helps you unlock. This often-overlooked technique can dramatically boost your strength, power, and muscle activation, making you a more explosive force in the ring.

This method acts as the link between strength and speed, training your muscles to produce maximum force on demand. It increases how quickly your muscles fire and apply force, meaning your body learns to apply strength more quickly, exactly what you need before moving into explosive plyometric work. Bruce Lee, known for his incredible speed and explosive power, was a big advocate of isometric training. He used it to build his legendary strength by focusing on generating maximum tension in his muscles. Lee used this method to teach his muscles to generate maximum force by pushing or pulling against immovable objects. The result? Explosive power and better muscle coordination.

Note: In this chapter, when we refer to isometrics, we're specifically talking about overcoming isometrics: maximal pushes or pulls against an immovable object. This is different from yielding isometrics (holding a weight in place), which serve other purposes.

Why Overcoming Isometrics Matter for Boxers

When it comes to striking, power goes beyond muscle. It's about the speed and efficiency with which you generate force. Overcoming isometrics train your body to deliver maximum effort instantly, making your punches faster, harder, and more explosive. By engaging fast-twitch muscle fibers, you prime your body to unleash force when it counts, whether throwing a knockout punch or holding your ground under pressure.

Isometric training does more than build strength; it conditions your body to deliver power on demand. When you punch, there's no time to gradually build strength. You need to generate maximum force instantly. This method sharpens your ability to do so with less effort and greater efficiency, while also improving coordination and reaction time. As a result, you'll be able to respond faster and seize openings the moment they appear, essential in a sport where every split second counts.

In addition to boosting explosive power, overcoming isometrics strengthen your tendons and stabilizer muscles, reducing injury risk and helping you absorb force more efficiently during a fight.

How to Incorporate Isometrics into Your Training

To get the most out of this training method, integrate them into your routine at least once per week, alongside your regular strength or boxing workouts. These exercises can be performed before a strength session to prime your muscles or as part of your conditioning routine.

Frequency: 1-3 times per week.

Sets: Start with 1-2 sets per exercise and gradually increase to 2-3 sets as your strength improves.

Fatigue Management: Overcoming isometrics are quick to perform and don't require much equipment, so you can easily fit them into your weekly training. They won't overload your muscles, but they will sharpen your strength and explosiveness. However, the neural demand is high, so use short efforts and keep total volume modest.

Time Under Tension Tip:

- **3-6 seconds:** Best for building raw explosive strength and speed. These short, intense efforts help sharpen your knockout power.

- **6-10 seconds:** Trains your ability to sustain power. This is ideal for finishing combinations or staying strong during explosive exchanges.

- **10-30 seconds:** Builds isometric endurance. Useful for clinch work, maintaining posture, and absorbing pressure when fatigued.

When to Use Isometrics

During off-season: Overcoming isometrics should be used alongside strength training to maximize force output and prepare for more explosive work.

During fight camp: The volume should be reduced, keeping intensity high but total work low, ensuring that strength is maintained without adding fatigue.

Before plyometric sessions: Performing a few sets of overcoming isometrics before plyos can prime the nervous system for maximum explosiveness.

Allow 48–72 hours before repeating heavy overcoming isometrics for the same joint angles.

Isometric Exercises for Boxers

These isometric exercises are designed to boost the specific muscles and movements needed for boxing. Each one targets key areas of strength and power generation:

Isometric Wall Push

How to Do It: Stand facing a wall with your hands at shoulder height. Push against the wall with maximum effort for 6-10 seconds, engaging your chest, shoulders, and triceps.

Focus: Boosts upper body strength and improves muscle activation, helping you stay powerful throughout the fight.

Isometric Punch Against Wall

How to Do It: Get into your boxing stance and carefully press your fist into the wall with controlled force, holding the position for six to 10 seconds. If your knuckles aren't conditioned, you can perform the hold using your palm while keeping your arm in punch position.

Jab: Use your lead hand to focus on speed and precision.

Cross: Drive power from your hips and shoulders.

Hook & Uppercut: Engage your entire torso and legs to deliver maximum force.

Focus: Builds raw punching strength and helps you generate force quickly and efficiently, training your body to release power on demand.

Isometric Deadlift Pull

How to Do It: Stand in a deadlift position and pull upwards on a barbell fixed at shin height, pulling with full effort for six to 10 seconds.

Focus: Strengthens your legs and back, both crucial for delivering powerful punches and maintaining balance during intense exchanges.

Isometric Shoulder Press

How to Do It: Press a fixed barbell upwards with maximum effort for 6 to 10 seconds, fully engaging your shoulders and triceps.

Focus: Develops upper body strength, especially in the shoulders and arms, essential for delivering strong punches and keeping your guard high.

Isometric Squats

How to Do It: Push against a barbell fixed in a squat position, pressing upwards with full force for 6 to 10 seconds.

Focus: Strengthens your legs, enhancing balance and power from the ground, which is key to generating force in your punches.

Safety Tips

Overcoming isometrics can deliver rapid strength gains, but they must be done safely to avoid injury:

- **Warm-Up First:** Start with a dynamic warm-up to get blood flowing to your muscles and joints.

- **Focus on Form:** Pay attention to posture and alignment, especially in your shoulders, back, and knees. Avoid straining joints by maintaining proper form throughout each exercise.

- **Cool-Down:** After each session, stretch your shoulders, legs, and back to prevent stiffness and maintain flexibility.

- **Breathe:** Avoid prolonged breath holds.

Adding Isometrics to Your Routine

By including this technique in your training, you'll build serious strength. These exercises don't take much time and require minimal equipment, making them easy to add to your weekly schedule.

As you progress, you'll notice increased force in your punches, leading to improved overall performance in the ring. You'll also feel stronger in clinch situations and more stable when absorbing impact, giving you greater control over the fight.

Each phase of training builds on the last. Core stability lays the groundwork for balance and control, calisthenics and light weights develop muscular endurance, and strength training builds the raw force needed for power. Olympic lifts help build strength with speed, and overcoming isometrics train your body to access that force instantly. But in a fight, you need to apply that force dynamically, repeatedly, and under pressure. That's where plyometrics and functional training complete the equation, bridging the gap between raw power and real-time explosiveness.

Chapter 30
Plyometrics: Explosive Power Unleashed

Plyometrics is all about developing ballistic power, speed, and quick reactions, qualities every boxer needs. Exercises like box jumps, clapping push-ups, and burpees help you generate explosive force in a short amount of time, for fast punches and dynamic footwork.

Beyond power, plyometrics also increase power endurance, the ability to sustain repeated bursts of high-intensity movement throughout a fight. This way you can stay dynamic from the first round to the last.

While plyometric training focuses on rapid, high-velocity movements like jumps and reactive drills, functional exercises provide a different kind of force-driven strength, one that transfers directly to fight-specific movements. These exercises condition your body to generate force dynamically, helping you apply power repeatedly and efficiently in real-world fight scenarios.

Functional movements, such as hammering a tire, chopping wood, kettlebell swings, landmine rotations, and weighted sled pushes, build power in ways that nicely translate to boxing. These exercises condition your body for the explosive actions needed to apply pressure, stay mobile, and deliver powerful punches.

Examples of Plyometric and Functional Exercises

Here are some examples of plyometric and functional exercises that can increase your fast-twitch power, endurance, and overall performance:

Alternating Jumping Lunges: Builds quick-twitch leg power, sharpens coordination, and strengthens your core to help you stay balanced and quick during changes in direction.

Box Jumps: Develops dynamic leg strength and agility, key for fast, controlled footwork.

Clapping Push-Ups: Increases upper body snap speed, helping you throw faster, more powerful punches.

Burpees: Combines full-body strength, cardio, and rapid-fire motion, improving endurance for repeated high-intensity movements.

Medicine Ball Slams: Develops core strength and upper-body drive, helping you generate downward power and engage your entire body in powerful movements.

Landmine Rotations: Builds rotational core power, for generating force in hooks and uppercuts, and enhances overall torso stability.

Weighted Sled Pushes: Enhances leg drive and endurance, crucial for maintaining pressure in the ring. This exercise is especially useful in close-range and inside fighting, where strong legs help you push your opponent back and control space.

Kettlebell Swings: Builds hip-driven power, strengthens your core, and enhances grip strength, making it excellent for boosting punching power and overall athleticism.

Hammering on a Tire: Develops upper-body strength and endurance, useful for maintaining power in sustained exchanges.

Chopping Wood: Strengthens your rotational core muscles and grip, increasing the power behind hooks and uppercuts.

Rotational Medicine Ball Throws: Enhances rotational power in your core, translating into stronger, more torque-driven punches.

Clarifying the Difference

While there's some overlap between movements, plyometric routines are generally structured for force-focused power development with full rest between sets, allowing your nervous system to fire at maximum intensity.

In contrast, explosive circuits are designed to simulate fight conditions, blending dynamic drills with continuous movement and minimal rest. Plyometrics build your raw firepower. Conditioning circuits train you to unleash it repeatedly when tired.

Sample Plyometrics Routine (Power Development Focus)

This routine uses lower volume and full recovery between sets. The goal is *maximum output* on every rep, train like a sprinter, not a marathoner.

- **Box Jumps:** 3 sets of 6 reps.
- **Clapping Push-Ups:** 2 sets of 6 reps.
- **Burpees:** 2 sets of 8 reps
- **Kettlebell Swings:** 3 sets of 10 reps.
- **Medicine Ball Slams:** 3 sets of 8 reps.
- (Full rest between sets)

Sample Conditioning Circuits (Power Under Fatigue)

These circuits simulate fight pace by combining high-effort movements with limited rest, conditioning your body to maintain power deep into demanding rounds.

Circuit Option 1: Explosive Power & Speed

3-4 rounds, 30 seconds work / 15 seconds rest per station.

1. **Box Jumps** (continuous)
2. **Clapping Push-Ups**
3. **Medicine Ball Slams**
4. **Alternating Jumping Lunges**
5. **Rotational Medicine Ball Throws**

Circuit Option 2: Functional Power & Fight-Specific Strength

3-4 rounds, 30 seconds work / 15 seconds rest per station.

1. **Hammer on Tire**
2. **Kettlebell Swings** (moderate weight)
3. **Landmine Rotations**
4. **Weighted Sled Pushes**

Safety Reminder

Plyometric and functional exercises are highly effective but physically demanding. Always prioritize form and control to prevent injury, as these rapid movements can strain your joints if done incorrectly. Start with lighter loads and shorter distances, gradually increasing intensity as your conditioning improves. Make sure you properly warm up before performing these exercises to prepare your muscles and joints for the dynamic movements ahead. Functional movements like chopping wood, hammering a tire, and kettlebell swings require solid technique to avoid injury, so focus on proper execution before increasing intensity.

Fight-Ready Conditioning: Sustaining Power Under Fatigue

Power is only useful if you can sustain it across multiple rounds. To keep your output high under strain, fighters can incorporate circuits that blend strength and endurance while maintaining potent delivery. These circuits aren't part of the structured periodization but serve as a great supplemental tool for fight preparation.

While traditional periodization structures neuromuscular training in dedicated phases, fighters can also benefit from doing circuits that blend power, endurance, and strength in a more fight-specific way. These circuits don't replace structured mesocycles but can be used to fine-tune power endurance in camp or as a maintenance strategy between fights.

By combining fast-force plyometric exercises with calisthenics and weighted movements like pull-ups, dips, and dumbbell snatches, these circuits condition the body to sustain repetitive strength bursts over multiple rounds. For fighters who want to improve their ability to preserve their punching power while taxed, the following circuits provide a strategic way to push endurance without sacrificing impact output.

Sample Fight-Ready Circuit (Explosive + Strength) – 3-Minute Rounds

Perform the following exercises continuously for 3 minutes, cycling through them as many times as possible.

Rest for 60 seconds, then repeat for 3-5 rounds.

6 Clapping Push-Ups *(quick-twitch upper-body force)*

6 Pull-Ups *(controlled upper-body strength)*

8 Box Jumps *(lower-body explosiveness & footwork)*

10-15 Dips *(upper-body endurance for extended power)*

6 Dumbbell Snatches (each side) *(full-body explosiveness)*

8 Medicine Ball Slams *(core-driven force)*

Customize Your Circuit

Fighters can mix and match any plyometric, functional, calisthenics, or dumbbell exercises to create circuits that fit their specific needs. Whether focusing on upper-body explosiveness, rotational power, or full-body endurance, the key is to keep movements dynamic and challenge you to keep going for the full round.

You've built the firepower. Now it's time to fuel the engine that keeps it burning.

Round 6: Endurance & Conditioning

Chapter 31
Cardiovascular Training

Boxing takes serious gas in the tank. You're not simply throwing punches, you're pushing your body to the limit, round after round. To keep that pace, you need a strong engine. Building your cardio improves how your body delivers oxygen, boosts endurance, and helps you recover quickly between exchanges. Running, swimming, and cycling are all solid tools to build the stamina it takes to perform at your best.

Why Cardiovascular Fitness Matters in Boxing

Energy and Endurance

Cardio training keeps your muscles fueled so you don't fade early. Steady-state runs build the kind of deep stamina that carries you through tough fights. Sprint intervals, hill runs, and stairs train you to fire off explosive bursts and recover fast, just like during real exchanges. Cycling adds variety and helps you stay strong during extended output. But nothing replaces roadwork. It's been a cornerstone of champions routines for a reason. It sharpens your body, your lungs, and your mindset.

Improved Recovery

Aerobic activities like steady-state runs help lower your heart rate and clear lactic acid, the stuff that builds up and makes your muscles burn, during breaks between rounds, allowing faster recovery. HIIT (high intensity interval training)-like sprints prepare you for the quick bursts of action and brief rest periods that reflect the rhythm of a fight, making sure you're ready for every exchange.

Swimming for Breath Control

Swimming offers unique cardiovascular benefits by improving lung capacity and breath control—both critical during high-pressure exchanges. It enhances oxygen efficiency while providing full-body conditioning with minimal impact on your joints, making it an excellent option for both cardio training and recovery.

Chapter 32
Running: The Essential Roadwork

Boxing's no fun if you don't run! It's a phrase that rings true for anyone who's spent hours pounding the pavement in preparation for the ring. There's a reason running remains one of the most time-tested methods in fight preparation. It's vital for building endurance, enhancing aerobic capacity, and improving cardiovascular health. The greats of old emphasized the importance of "roadwork", and even with modern advances in sports science, running—whether long-duration (aerobic) or high-intensity sprints (anaerobic), see chapter 23— remains one of the best tools for conditioning a fighter. Skipping this important piece of training can leave you underprepared for the stamina required in the ring.

When you run, you're doing more than just logging miles. Roadwork, particularly longer-duration running, improves your body's ability to transport oxygen to your muscles, allowing you to push yourself harder and longer before fatigue sets in. Today this is often overlooked, believing boxing is purely a fast-twitch, high intensity sport. But without a strong aerobic base, fast-twitch muscles burn out quickly, leaving fighters exhausted after just a few rounds. Sustained aerobic running strengthens your heart, lungs, and improves blood flow to your muscles, ensuring your body can repeatedly fuel explosive movements over an entire fight. Fighters with great anaerobic bursts but poor aerobic endurance often gas out when their power output can't be sustained.

At the same time, sprint work enhances explosive power and conditions your body to tolerate high-intensity efforts, while a strong aerobic base helps you recover faster between bursts. Both forms of running help build strength endurance in your legs, which is crucial for maintaining agility and footwork throughout a fight.

What Makes Running So Effective?

Endurance and Energy: Running increases the number of mitochondria (the "powerhouse" of your cells), enabling your muscles to generate sustained energy. In simple terms, it gives you the staying power to keep fighting when the rounds stack up.

Quicker Recovery: Roadwork improves how efficiently your body recovers between explosive bursts. Longer-duration roadwork builds endurance to help you catch your breath faster between exchanges, while interval sprints train your ability to sustain explosive output and tolerate fatigue during high-intensity moments in the fight.

Footwork and Agility: Strong legs are the foundation of great movement. Roadwork strengthens your lower body, ensuring you can pivot, shuffle, and create angles effortlessly throughout a fight.

Mental Resilience: Running mile after mile pushes you past physical and mental limits, teaching you to embrace discomfort. This grit translates directly to the ring, where the mentally tough often prevail. Long runs are also one of the best times for visualization. Mentally rehearsing the fight, picturing success, and narrowing focus while the body is in motion. At the same time, they serve a practical role in keeping weight under control, making roadwork not just a conditioning tool but a strategic one.

Elite Boxers Who Run

Historically, running has been fundamental to the training of the sport's greatest champions. Sugar Ray Robinson credited his roadwork with helping him stay light on his feet and maintain the rhythm and fluidity that defined his performances. He believed running gave him the endurance to sustain his rapid combinations and agile footwork, allowing him to control the fight from start to finish.

Marvin Hagler, another all-time great, famously incorporated backward running into his routine, running at least one mile in reverse during his roadwork. This unconventional technique helped improve his coordination, balance, and ability to move backward defensively while boxing.

In the modern boxing landscape, fighters continue to value the endurance-building effects of running. David Benavidez, known for his relentless pressure and ability to *turn up the heat* in the championship rounds, also emphasizes long-distance running during his training camps. This allows him to keep pushing the pace and wear down his opponents over multiple rounds.

Meanwhile, sprint training has also gained prominence. Fighters like Naoya Inoue and Gervonta Davis focus on explosive sprints to build quickness and lower-body power. Whether it's stair sprints or resistance sprints using parachutes and bands, these intense bursts of speed training simulate the fast-twitch movements needed for explosive punches and quick transitions in the ring.

A Tailored Approach to Running

Not all runs are created equal. By varying your roadwork, you can target different aspects of your conditioning, from explosive power to sustained endurance. Here's how to customize your training:`

Endurance Building

Longer-Duration Running: Build stamina and cardiovascular endurance with steady-state runs. Extended runs help fend off fatigue and maintain a strong performance throughout the fight. The right pace should feel steady but sustainable — you should be able to hold a conversation without gasping for air (Zone 2 heart rate).

Example: Run for 30-90 minutes at a moderate pace.

Frequency: 2–4 sessions per week is ideal in camp. Early on, lean toward the higher end (3–4 runs) to build your aerobic base; later in camp, scale back to 1–2 runs while adding more sprint and interval work.

Fartlek Running: With unstructured tempo changes, fartlek running improves your ability to adapt to different fight rhythms, switching between fast-paced exchanges and measured pacing.

Example: Run at a moderate pace for 3 minutes, then sprint for 1 minute, jog for 2 minutes, and repeat for 30 minutes.

Explosive Power

Interval Running: Mimicking the dynamics of a boxing match, interval running helps you develop explosive power and speed, followed by brief recovery periods.

Example: After a warm-up, sprint for 30 seconds, jog for 1 minute. Repeat for 20 minutes.

Hill Running: Running up hills strengthens your legs and builds the driving force needed to maintain pressure during a fight.

Example: After a warm-up, sprint uphill for 30 seconds, walk back down. Repeat 10-15 times.

Bridge Runs: Long bridge inclines combine the benefits of steady roadwork with resistance training, forcing your legs, lungs, and heart to work harder over an extended stretch. They build endurance under load while building the mental toughness needed for championship rounds.

Example: Run the length of a bridge at a steady pace on the incline, maintain form across the descent, and repeat for 30–45 minutes.

Stair Sprints: Build lower-body spring and reactivity, expand your lungs, and improve your ability 1to quickly move in and out of range.

Example: After a warm-up, sprint up a flight of stairs for 20 seconds, walk down, and repeat for 10-15 rounds.

Treadmill Sprints: If you prefer indoor training or want a controlled environment, treadmill sprints are a great option. You can adjust the incline to make the workout more challenging or use speed intervals to build burst power and quickness.

Example: After a warm-up, sprint for 30 seconds, then walk or jog for 1 minute. Repeat for 15 minutes.

Agility and Coordination

Trail Running: Running on uneven terrain builds strength, balance, and coordination, simulating the need for strong footwork and stability in the ring.

Example: Run on a forest trail for 30-60 minutes.

Retro Running (popularized by Marvin Hagler): Running backward engages different muscle groups and improves your ability to move in reverse—building leg endurance for fighting while retreating.

Example: Run backward for 1 minute, jog forward for 1 minute. Repeat for 20 minutes.

Sand Running: Running on sand builds explosive power in your legs while improving balance, coordination, and agility.

Example: Run on a beach for 30-45 minutes, incorporating sprints and lateral movements.

The Road to Victory

Running is an indispensable part of your training, delivering both physical and mental benefits that directly enhance your performance in the ring. Whether you're building endurance with steady-state roadwork or developing explosiveness with interval sprints, running helps build the stamina, strength, and mental toughness needed to conquer your opponents. So, lace up your shoes, hit the pavement, and take control of your journey to greatness, because every mile you run brings you one step closer to victory.

Chapter 33
Aquatic Training: Unlocking Superhuman Stamina

Swimming is a low-impact, full-body workout with serious benefits for boxers. It boosts your cardio, builds muscular endurance, and helps you recover faster. Roadwork will always be the foundation of a boxer's conditioning, but swimming is a powerful addition: giving you performance gains without pounding your joints. Adding water-based training to your routine gives your body relief while still challenging your limits.

Benefits of Swimming for Boxers

Increased Cardiovascular Fitness: Swimming puts your heart and lungs to the test, significantly enhancing your endurance. The natural resistance of the water makes every stroke count, building the stamina you need to maintain peak energy during a fight.

Increased Lung Capacity: The controlled breathing in swimming trains you to manage your breath better, expanding your lung capacity. That means better oxygen control when the pace picks up and you're deep in the fight, where every breath matters.

Muscular Endurance and Strength: Swimming hits multiple muscle groups at once, building full-body strength and endurance without the impact stress of land-based exercises. The constant resistance builds a balanced, powerful physique while lowering the risk of overuse injuries.

Recovery and Rehabilitation: The buoyancy of water takes pressure off your joints and muscles, making it perfect for active recovery. You can keep your fitness up while giving your body a break from the grind of daily boxing training.

Elite Boxers Who Swim

Beyond these physical benefits, let's explore how elite boxers are harnessing the power of water to sharpen their performance.

Vasyl Lomachenko and Oleksandr Usyk: Both elite fighters integrate swimming into their routines to improve endurance and agility, leveraging the physical and mental benefits of aquatic training.

Terence Crawford: Crawford uses swimming to build endurance and recover quickly. His ability to maintain energy between rounds is a testament to his dedication to aquatic training.

Jermell Charlo: Swimming boosts Charlo's cardiovascular endurance and overall fitness, helping him maintain high energy levels throughout his fights.

Juan Diaz: Known for his relentless style, Diaz used swimming to maintain the stamina needed for a high punch output, allowing him to push through long, grueling fights.

Putting Swimming into Your Training

Schedule Regular Sessions: Aim for one or two swimming sessions per week to gain cardiovascular and muscular benefits without overloading your training schedule.

Focus on Technique: Proper technique is key to maximizing results and preventing injury. Consider working with a swimming coach to ensure your form is efficient and effective.

Mix Up Your Workouts: Alternate between different strokes and intensities to engage various muscle groups and keep your workouts challenging.

Interval Training in Water: Do high-intensity intervals followed by recovery periods to mimic the intensity of boxing rounds. This helps improve your cardiovascular endurance and stamina for the ring.

Underwater Punching Drills: Punching underwater while standing shoulder-deep strengthens your punches by adding resistance. This drill develops arm and shoulder endurance, improves breath control during extended exchanges in the ring, and enhances overall conditioning. Fully submerged, underwater punching and swimming also improve your CO_2 tolerance, further boosting your endurance.

Use Swimming for Recovery: You can also use swimming as a tool for active recovery. It's ideal for low-impact conditioning when your muscles and joints need a break from the rigors of regular boxing training.

Harnessing the Power of Water

Swimming is more than just a workout. It takes your conditioning to another level, setting you apart in the ring. Whether you're aiming to enhance your cardiovascular fitness, improve lung capacity, or speed up recovery, adding aquatic training to your regimen can boost stamina and give you an edge in the ring. Dive in, harness the power of water, and unlock a new level of conditioning that few fighters tap into.

Chapter 34
Pedal Power: Strengthening Leg Stamina

Cycling is a powerful tool for boosting cardio and building leg endurance in boxing. It brings several key benefits to the table, making it a smart addition to your training routine. Whether you're trying to level up your conditioning, increase balance, strengthen your legs, or sharpen your mental edge, cycling delivers.

Like swimming, cycling offers a great way to build stamina, improve cardiovascular health, and minimize joint strain. It's the perfect complement to roadwork, offering serious conditioning without the high-impact stress of running.

Benefits of Cycling for Boxers

Joint-Friendly Conditioning: Cycling builds endurance and leg strength in a way that you can sustain throughout a full camp, without the wear and tear of constant pavement runs.

Versatile Workouts: You can tailor your rides however you want. Long, steady rides for stamina, or short, explosive intervals that mimic the rhythm of a fight.

Stronger Legs for Boxing: Stronger legs mean sharper movement, and more stamina. Regular cycling builds the kind of leg endurance that keeps you mobile and powerful from round one to the final bell.

Better Cardio Health: It boosts heart and lung function, helping you recover faster between rounds and stay energized deep into a fight.

Improved Balance: Cycling enhances your body's ability to stabilize, especially as you work on pedaling while maintaining posture. This translates to better overall balance in the ring.

Mental Toughness: Long rides and intense intervals build that inner grit, training your mind to keep going when your body wants to quit.

Adding the Airdyne Bike

The Airdyne bike, a stationary bike with moving handlebars, turns up the intensity. The harder you pedal, the more resistance you face, mimicking the kind of explosive effort boxing demands. Its dual-action motion works both your upper and lower body at the same time, improving endurance and coordination in one shot.

Sample Airdyne Workout

- **Warm-up:** 5 minutes of moderate effort.
- **Intervals**: Sprint for 30 seconds while pumping your arms, then pedal and move your arms slowly for 90 seconds. Repeat for 8-10 rounds.
- **Cool-down:** 5 minutes of light pedaling and arm movement.

Elite Boxers Who Cycle

Former middleweight champ Sergio Martinez used cycling to build insane stamina and maintain high energy in the ring. Mike Tyson also incorporated stationary bike work as part of his cool-down routine, strengthening his legs and aiding recovery while maintaining the endurance that made him dangerous even late into fights.

How to Add Cycling to Your Training

There are different ways to use cycling to improve your boxing performance:

- **High-Intensity Interval Training (HIIT)**: Sprint for 30 seconds, recover for 1 minute with slow pedaling. Do this for 20–30 minutes to replicate fight bursts and recovery.

- **Endurance Rides**: Go at a steady pace for 45–90 minutes. These rides build deep stamina and strong legs for long fights.

- **Recovery Rides**: On off days, hop on the bike for 30–45 minutes at a light pace. You'll keep blood flowing and help your body bounce back without adding more stress.

Frequency: Aim for 2–3 cycling sessions per week, depending on your needs in camp. Treat it as a complement to roadwork. It's great for recovery days, endurance boosts, or interval sharpening, without replacing your runs entirely.

Other Low-Impact Options

While running, cycling, and swimming are the core conditioning methods for fighters, other tools like the elliptical, rowing machine, or assault bike can offer variety, especially for recovery days or fighters rehabbing injuries. These machines still improve cardiovascular output, but they're best used to supplement, not replace, your main roadwork.

Chapter 35
Overlooked and Uncommon Methods for Elite Physical Conditioning & Performance

If you've made it this far, you're already way ahead of the curve. Not every method in this section will apply to you right now, but the serious ones will keep these in their back pocket and pull the right tools at the right time. This chapter isn't here to overwhelm you. It's here to sharpen the blade. This is about building out the parts of your body most fighters ignore. So study the details. Then weaponize them.

To reach the highest levels, a fighter has to be built for war, capable of dishing out damage, taking it, and staying dangerous deep into the fight. That kind of durability doesn't come from basic training. It comes from smart, targeted methods that forge real-world toughness. Ones that strengthen your body in all the right places, increase your conditioning, and harden you against the grind of combat.

Some of these methods are advanced. Others are just underused. The goal? Build a fighter who's still throwing heat when others are falling apart.

What You'll Learn in This Section

- **Dynamic Resistance Training:** Utilizing weighted vests, resistance bands, and contrast training to enhance speed, power, and endurance.

- **Building Stronger Forearms, Hands, and Wrists:** Developing grip strength, durability, and impact resistance to increase punch effectiveness.

- **Breathing Techniques for Endurance and Stamina:** Training the lungs and oxygen efficiency to push beyond fatigue and maintain composure under pressure.

- **Enhancing Punch Resistance:** Strengthening the neck, core, and body for superior punch absorption and injury prevention.
- **Stretching & Mobility for Boxers:** Enhancing fluidity, recovery, and injury prevention with dynamic and static mobility drills.

Each of these areas plays a vital role in maximizing performance, whether it's developing knockout power, taking body shots without folding, or ensuring your endurance never fades in the later rounds. By integrating these methods into your routine, you will build the ultimate fighter's body: one that delivers punishment just as well as it endures it.

Dynamic Resistance Training— Powering Up Your Boxing Performance

Picture yourself throwing punches with the power of a heavyweight, while still moving with the effortless speed of a lightweight. Dynamic resistance training can bring this to life, shaping your body into a finely tuned weapon. Push your limits with weighted vests, hand weights, ankle weights, and resistance bands. Each tool forces your body to adapt, unlocking new levels of strength, speed, and endurance.

Even if you've never watched *Dragon Ball Z*, imagine warriors pushing their limits by training with weighted clothing. In the famous anime, Goku and his friends wore weighted gear to grow stronger, then shed it to unleash their full power. You can apply the same principle in your training. By using resistance tools and then removing them, you'll move lighter, faster, and more explosively, just like shedding armor and revealing the weapon beneath.

Benefits of Dynamic Resistance Training

Enhanced Punching Power: Adding resistance with tools like weighted vests, hand weights, or resistance bands forces your muscles to work harder. This extra effort builds strength and endurance, leading to stronger, more powerful punches over time.

Improved Agility and Speed: Resistance training challenges your muscles to generate more force during movement, which enhances your coordination and explosiveness. Over time, this leads to quicker, more dynamic footwork and faster, more impactful punches.

Boosted Cardiovascular Fitness: Training with added weight challenges your muscles, your heart and lungs. This extra strain builds stamina, so when you don't have the resistance, you can go longer and harder without tiring as quickly.

Strengthened Core and Stability: The added load from resistance gear forces your core muscles to work harder, improving your overall balance and stability. As a result, you'll maintain better control during training and develop the endurance to withstand tough rounds.

Leveraging Dynamic Resistance for Maximum Impact

Weighted Vests: Wear a weighted vest (typically 5-20 lbs) during shadowboxing, footwork drills, or jump rope. Start with a lighter weight to get comfortable with the added resistance. The extra load pushes your muscles and cardiovascular system to work harder, building more power and endurance over time. For an even greater challenge, pair the vest with ankle or hand weights.

Hand Weights: Use 1-5 pound hand weights during shadowboxing. These help build shoulder endurance, allowing you to keep up a higher punch output without tiring as quickly. Over time, your punches will stay sharp and consistent, even in later rounds.

Ankle Weights: Add ankle weights (1-5 pounds per leg) to shadowboxing, skipping, or footwork drills. Start with a lighter weight if you're new to ankle weights, and increase as needed based on your comfort. This extra resistance strengthens your legs, improving the efficiency and control of your footwork, making your movements quicker and more precise.

Resistance Bands: Hold the ends of a resistance band in each hand and loop the band around your back. This creates tension that forces your core and upper body to work harder with every punch. Adjust the tension by choosing different bands or tightening them for a greater challenge.

Contrast Training: Supercharge Your Results

Contrast training takes dynamic resistance to the next level by alternating between exercises with and without weighted gear. This method allows you to take advantage of a temporary boost in speed and agility, making your body move quicker and more explosively. As you consistently train this way, your body adapts, learning to move faster and feel lighter naturally, even without the additional weight.

Putting Contrast Training into Practice

Here's how you can start adding resistance tools to your workouts for maximum effect.

Weighted Vest and Shadowboxing: Start with a weighted vest for 3 rounds of shadowboxing. When the vest comes off, your entire body will feel lighter, and your movements will feel quicker and smoother.

Hand Weights and Shadowboxing: Shadowbox with light hand weights for a few rounds. After you put the weights down, your punches will feel faster, with a noticeable increase in speed.

Ankle Weights and Footwork Drills: Perform footwork drills with ankle weights. After removing them, your legs will feel lighter, making your steps faster and more responsive.

Resistance Bands and Punching Drills: Use resistance bands to throw punches for a few rounds, focusing on maintaining speed and form. After removing the bands, throw unresisted punches. Some may feel an increase in speed due to reduced resistance, while others may primarily notice improved endurance and control.

Note: For an even greater effect, try using a weighted vest, hand weights, and ankle weights together. When you remove all three, your entire body will feel significantly lighter, allowing you to move with enhanced ability.

Strength-Based PAP Drills for Explosive Power

Another way to build quick-twitch power in your punches is through Post-Activation Potentiation (PAP). This method trains your muscles to fire faster and harder by pairing a heavy strength exercise with an explosive movement that uses the same muscles.

Think of it like waking up your muscles with a heavy lift so they work at full capacity when you switch to a fast, powerful movement. Over time, this helps your punches feel sharper, your footwork feel quicker, and your movements feel more effortless in the ring.

Here's how to put it to work:

Heavy Dumbbell Chest Press → Explosive Push-Ups

→ Press heavy dumbbells for 5-8 reps to activate your upper body strength.
→ Immediately drop down for 5-10 explosive push-ups, pushing off the ground with power.
→ Afterward, throw a few fast, crisp punches—just enough to feel the increased speed and snap.

Heavy Squats → Jump Squats

→ Perform 3-8 heavy squats to load your legs with strength.

→ Follow it up with 5-10 jump squats, exploding off the ground.

Trap Bar Deadlifts → Broad Jumps

→ Lift heavy with a trap bar deadlift for 3-8 reps to engage your entire lower body.

→ Immediately do 5 broad jumps, covering as much distance as possible.

→ You'll feel the extra explosiveness in your legs when stepping into punches or shifting your weight.

Heavy Dumbbell One-Arm Rear Delt Row → Australian Pull-Ups

→ Perform 5-8 heavy one-arm rear delt rows per side, keeping your movements powerful and controlled.

→ Immediately move to Australian pull-ups (bodyweight rows):

- o Find a sturdy bar or rings at waist height.
- o Lie under it with your feet extended in front of you and your body in a straight line.
- o Grip the bar and pull your chest up while keeping your core tight.
- o Lower under control, then explode back up for 5-10 reps, focusing on speed.
- o Make sure to pull explosively, this will train your rear delts and back to retract punches faster.

How to Use PAP Training

Add these drills one or two times a week as part of your strength training. After doing the PAP exercises, throw a few fast punches, enough to feel the increased speed and snap so your body registers the improvement.

Over time, your body will adapt and make these gains permanent, helping you punch harder, move quicker, and react faster in real fights. Master this, and you'll hit with the kind of speed and force that fighters feel...but can't explain.

Building Stronger Forearms, Hands, and Wrists for Boxing

Punch power, precision, and control are hallmarks of a great boxer, but behind every solid shot lies a set of often-overlooked muscles that can give you that "heavy hands" effect, turning every punch into a brick. In this chapter, we'll break down why forearms, wrists, hands, and even fingers matter, and how to train them for knockout stability and power.

Power Transfer and Punch Stability

A solid forearm and wrist act like a bridge, channeling energy from your body to your opponent. Without that strength, punches lose power on impact; with it, they land with an undeniable force. Forearm strength helps fighters keep their fists steady, allowing punches to hit with bone-crushing authority. Strong forearms can leave opponents rocked and reeling, each punch landing with the kind of precision and intensity that makes an impact, and a statement.

Protecting Your Greatest Assets

Your hands are your primary weapons in the ring. Boxing's relentless strain on the small bones and joints in the hands and wrists can lead to injuries that sideline fighters, sometimes for months or longer (as I know all too well). A routine focused on forearm and wrist stability doesn't just protect your hands from injury—it builds a layer of resilience, making you less vulnerable to sprains and strains and keeping you in the game longer.

Exercises for Brute Forearm and Grip Strength

The following exercises have been used by legends to build unmatched power and endurance in their hands and wrists. Add just one or two of these exercises at the end of your workouts or on strength-focused days, and watch your punch stability, grip, and command grow.

Forearm Grippers

The simplicity of forearm grippers belies their impact. Squeeze with all your strength, hold, then release, feeling the burn through your forearms. This builds crushing grip strength and relentless forearm power that translates directly into punching force. Aim for 3 sets of 10-15 squeezes, holding each squeeze for 3-5 seconds.

Kettlebell Wrist Rotations

A powerful tool, kettlebell wrist rotations work wonders for stability. Hold the kettlebell on its side, using wrist strength to rotate it back and forth. This movement develops the wrist control and grip authority that lets punches stay solid. Try 10-15 rotations each way.

Rice Bucket Training

Filling a bucket with rice, push your hands into the grains, opening and closing your fingers. Twist and press as you dig deeper, feeling the resistance build hand and finger power. This exercise also strengthens the forearms, reinforcing grip endurance and wrist stability, which translates to stronger, more controlled punches. It's a favorite among fighters who understand that hand strength begins in the smallest muscles, giving you a denser punch.

Wrist Rollers

Wrist rollers work through a full range of motion, building a sustained burn and resilience in the wrist and forearm that keeps punches rock solid. Roll up, then roll down for a controlled, powerful burn. Aim for 1-2 minutes each set.

Push-Ups on Fists and Fingers

A true test of toughness, fist and finger push-ups build wrist stability and knuckle durability, fortifying your hands for intense impact. For fighters ready for the challenge, finger push-ups add another layer of power. Start with 2-3 sets of 10-15 reps, and use fingers only if you've mastered the knuckle push-up.

Dead Hangs

Dead hangs from a pull-up bar develop raw finger strength and powerful grip endurance, critical for long rounds. Start with 20-30 seconds, adding time as you progress. Feel the tension and control build, helping punches stay firm and impactful.

> **Tip:** Don't try to do all of these at once. Choose 2-3 based on your needs and rotate them in at the end of your sessions or during strength days. A little consistency goes a long way.

Include these exercises into your regular strength workouts or at the end of your training sessions to build stronger forearms, hands, and wrists without overloading your routine.

Honoring the Legacy of Forearm and Grip Strength

Few fighters have demonstrated the transformative power of forearm strength like Bruce Lee. A fanatic for forearm conditioning, Lee believed that strong forearms could turn ordinary punches into knockout blows. He invented and refined tools, from wrist rollers to custom grip developers, to make his forearms a well of untapped power. Every strike became a lightning bolt of energy, amplified by the strength built in his hands and wrists.

Gennady Golovkin embodied this same intensity. Known for bone-rattling punches, Golovkin harnessed forearm power through kettlebell wrist rotations, among other methods, helping create a level of power in his strikes that commanded respect. This dedication to forearm training became part of his signature style, allowing him to leave opponents on the canvas, dazed and overwhelmed by the sheer force behind his hands.

The stronger your hands and wrists, the more weight you carry with every shot. Build them right, and your opponents won't just feel your power, they'll remember it.

The Oxygen Edge: Breath Training for Elite Endurance

When fatigue sets in for both combatants, the fighter who can push a little deeper and last a little longer gains a real advantage. Breath control won't magically fix bad conditioning, but it's one of those overlooked tools that can give you an edge when the fight gets tough.

Most fighters ignore breath training altogether, which is exactly why adding it to your routine can give you a serious advantage. Fighters like Vasyl Lomachenko and Oleksandr Usyk, known for their relentless pace, train their breathing just like they train their punches. They don't rely on raw conditioning alone. They sharpen every weapon, including the ability to manage oxygen and stay calm under fire.

By incorporating techniques like rhythmic breathing, breath-holding drills, and inspiratory muscle training, you can fine-tune your endurance, stay composed under pressure, and recover faster between exchanges. It won't replace hard conditioning, but it adds another layer to your arsenal that can make a real difference when everything else is equal.

How to Perform Rhythmic Breathing

Find your zone by sitting or lying down somewhere safe and comfortable, where you can focus fully. *Do* not do this while driving, standing, or mid-training.

Take 30 deep breaths, inhaling fully through your nose or mouth, then exhaling naturally without forcing all the air out. Keep a steady rhythm, each breath flowing into the next without pause. You might feel tingling, lightheaded, or warm—this is your body adjusting to shifts in oxygen and CO_2.

After the last exhale, take a deep inhale, hold for 15 seconds, then release naturally.

Repeat this process for as many rounds as you feel necessary to achieve a relaxed and focused state.

Why This Matters for Fighters: A quick round of rhythmic breathing before training or sparring can help you control tension, get into a relaxed but focused state, and improve breath efficiency. Used consistently, it helps you stay composed when breathing gets heavy, keeping your mind clear as rounds wear on.

Before using this before sparring, experiment with it during regular training to see how your body responds. Some fighters may feel lightheaded at first, while others adapt quickly.

Note: *Combining rhythmic breathing with short breath-holds (around 15 seconds) can be safely done before training or sparring, helping you stay calm and focused. Longer breath-holding drills, however, are best done after training. Post-workout, they condition your body to handle oxygen deprivation under fatigue, simulating late-fight exhaustion and improving recovery under stress.*

A full breakdown of breath-holding techniques and how to apply them is covered next.

Breath-Holding Exercises: Push Your Limits and Build Endurance

(CO2 Tolerance & Stress Adaptation)

Every fighter knows the feeling—lungs burning, muscles heavy, and your body begging for a breath. Whether you're trading in a high-volume exchange, grinding through the last rounds of a close fight, or defending under sustained pressure, breath control can mean the difference between staying on point or falling apart. Breath-holding drills help you handle these moments more effectively by improving CO2 tolerance, oxygen efficiency, and breath control under stress.

By forcing your body to adapt to lower oxygen levels, you'll learn to stay calm, keep your movement crisp, and outlast opponents who start to fade when the gas tank runs low.

Drills and Techniques to Improve CO2 Tolerance

Apnea—which means breath-holding—is used to train your body and mind to stay calm and perform under rising CO2 levels. These variations simulate fight pressure and help you recover your breathing more quickly between rounds or after explosive exchanges.

Static apnea builds CO2 tolerance and teaches you to stay relaxed as the urge to breathe intensifies. Hold your breath while seated or lying down, gradually increasing the time.

Walking apnea requires holding your breath while walking and gradually increasing the number of steps. This improves breath control and CO2 tolerance, but dynamic apnea is better for simulating fight conditions.

Dynamic apnea is the most fight *relevant*. Combining breath-holding with movements like short sprints, jump rope, or light footwork. This puts your body under low-oxygen stress in a safe way, simulating the fatigue and pressure you feel late in a round.

Breath counting helps regulate breathing after intense training and strengthens overall breath control. Inhale for 8 seconds, exhale for 10, and stretch the duration over time.

Box breathing helps calm nerves, manage adrenaline, and sharpen focus before fights or training. Inhale for 4 seconds, hold for 4, exhale for 4, hold for 4. Simple but effective..

Max breath-hold training is about pushing your absolute limit. For best results, do this after a full exhale, then hold your breath as long as possible to test endurance. This isn't structured training like static apnea—it's a way to gauge progress and build mental resilience. Push your limits and track progress weekly.

Tip: You'll be able to hold your breath for longer if you do rhythmic breathing first. Save intense holds for after training to replicate end-of-fight stress.

While breath-holding drills train your mind and body to function under oxygen stress, IMT focuses on strengthening the breathing muscles themselves. This is where you develop the raw hardware to breathe deeper, more efficiently, and under control. Especially in the later rounds.

Inspiratory Muscle Training (IMT): Strengthen Your Breathing Power

(Breathing Muscle Strength & Efficiency)

Stronger breathing muscles let you take in more air with less effort, helping you stay composed and recover faster as the fight wears on. Inspiratory Muscle Training (IMT) strengthens the muscles responsible for breathing, allowing you to maximize oxygen intake and breathe more efficiently under pressure. Specifically, it targets the inspiratory muscles—like the diaphragm and intercostals—which are responsible for pulling air into the lungs.

Why This Matters in Combat Sports: If your breathing stays controlled, your whole body remains sharper and more responsive. Stronger respiratory muscles make it easier to maintain pace under stress, preventing unnecessary fatigue. Better breath control also leads to faster recovery between exchanges.

Tools & Drills for IMT

Diaphragmatic breathing, also called "belly breathing", fully engages your diaphragm instead of relying on shallow chest breathing.

IMT devices like Threshold IMT or PowerLung add resistance to inhalation, forcing your breathing muscles to work harder.

Respiratory resistance masks build breathing muscle endurance but DO NOT simulate altitude training.

How to Use Breathing Resistance Masks Correctly

Start gradually with short sessions and low resistance—**don't overdo it.** These masks are not meant to be worn for the entire training session. Use them for specific rounds, drills, or short intervals to avoid overuse and strain on the lungs.

Monitor your breathing. If you feel lightheaded, reduce resistance and take breaks.

Cooldown without the mask to let your body reset before finishing training.

Boosting Blood Flow with Supplements

Looking for an extra boost? Some natural supplements help improve circulation, which can support endurance and recovery.

L-Citrulline boosts nitric oxide levels, improving blood flow and reducing muscle fatigue.

Beetroot powder is a natural source of nitrates, which widen blood vessels and improve endurance.

Cordyceps mushrooms are used by endurance athletes to support lung function and overall stamina.

These won't replace hard training, but they can help give you a little more gas in the tank when it counts.

Final Thoughts—Is This Worth It?

These breathing techniques won't turn a weak gas tank into elite endurance overnight, nor will the supplements. But for fighters looking to gain an edge, fine-tuning your breathing mechanics, CO_2 tolerance, and oxygen efficiency can make a real difference over time.

This is just one more way to separate yourself from opponents who only focus on the obvious training methods. The best fighters use every tool available, and breath training is one of those subtle but powerful weapons.

You've built your weapons. Powerful punches, relentless endurance, and the physical tools to push through war. But all of that means nothing if you can't hold up when it matters most.

Because in boxing you have to be able to *give* it... and you have to be able to *take* it.

Chapter 36
The Key to Taking Punches

Every fighter knows that no matter how good their defense is, they're going to get hit. What separates top fighters from the rest is their ability to withstand those punches, stay on their feet, and continue fighting. True resilience in the ring isn't about being tough. It's about being prepared.

Prepare for Impact: Neck Training

If you want to improve your punch resistance and develop a "good chin", neck training is non-negotiable. Building up the strength in your neck dramatically increases your ability to "take a punch". It acts as a shock absorber, reducing the risk of knockouts.

Fitness & Power of the Mind

Being in top physical shape is not purely about offense, it's key to taking punches too. A well-conditioned body can absorb shots better. Plain and simple. And if you're draining yourself with extreme weight cuts, you're setting yourself up to get rocked. Dehydration and lost strength make you way more vulnerable.

Mindset is just as important. Virgil Hunter (trainer of Andre Ward) said, "Part of taking a punch is mental. Make up your mind that no matter what they hit you with, you're not going anywhere." Marvin Hagler embodied this attitude when he said, "In order to knock me out, you better hit me with that ring post because I ain't going nowhere." A strong mental approach, combined with physical preparation, makes a fighter much harder to break.

Exemplary Fighters

Some of boxing's greatest fighters, like Canelo Alvarez, Gennady "GGG" Golovkin, and Mike Tyson, are known for their extraordinary punch resistance, a quality they attribute to rigorous neck training. They religiously worked on their neck muscles, which plays a significant role in their ability to withstand powerful blows and remain resilient in the ring.

The Importance of Neck Strength

When you take a punch to the head, the force causes your head to whiplash to the back or side, potentially leading to concussions or knockouts. A strong neck helps stabilize the head, absorb impact, and minimize the damage. It doesn't make you invincible, but it dramatically helps you take a better shot.

Neck Training for Boxers

To develop ironclad punch resistance, include these key neck exercises in your training regimen:

Neck Harness

How to Use It: Attach a neck harness to a weight and secure it around your head. Perform neck curls and extensions while seated or standing.

Why It Works: Directly strengthens the front, back, and sides of the neck, building overall stability.

Iron Neck Exercise Machine (or resistance bands as an alternative)

How to Use It: The Iron Neck allows for a full range of motion exercises; rotations, flexions, and extensions. If unavailable, use a resistance band around the head and perform similar movements.

Why It Works: Strengthens the neck in multiple directions, improving control and resistance to sudden impact.

Neck Curls

How to Do It: Lie on a bench or floor with your head hanging off the edge. Hold a weight plate on your forehead and lift your head toward your chest. Repeat with your head turned left, right, and facing down to strengthen all areas.

Why It Works: Targets all major neck muscles, improving resistance from multiple angles.

Side Neck Bridges

How to Do It: Lie on your side with your head resting on a firm but cushioned surface, such as a folded towel, a yoga mat, or a wrestling mat. Push your head into the surface, lifting your shoulders off the ground. Hold for a few seconds before lowering. If you're not yet able to lift your shoulders, start by pressing your head into the surface with pressure, to engage the muscles and gradually build up strength.

Why It Works: Strengthens side neck muscles, critical for minimizing lateral whiplash when hit.

Isometric Neck Exercises

How to Do It: Press your hand against your forehead and push your head against it without allowing any movement. Hold the tension for 10-15 seconds. Repeat by placing your hand on the back of your head and the sides.

Why It Works: Builds static strength, which is important for absorbing punches.

Front Neck Bridges (Modified for Safety)

How to Do It: Kneel on the floor with a Bosu ball positioned under your forehead. With your body in a push-up position, gently press your forehead into the Bosu ball, supporting your weight through your legs and core. Hold the position for a few seconds, then lower yourself back down.

Why It Works: Builds front neck strength while reducing strain on the spine.

Towel in Mouth with Kettlebell (Jaw & Neck Strength)

How to Use It: Loop a towel through the handle of a kettlebell, bringing the towel ends together. Stand or sit with a slight forward hinge at the waist. Bite down on the towel ends and lift the kettlebell by raising and lowering your head.

Why It Works: This exercise strengthens the jaw and neck muscles, improving overall punch resistance.

Silicone Jaw Strengthener

How to Use It: Place the silicone jaw strengthener in your mouth and bite down repeatedly. Start with 3 sets of 10-15 repetitions, gradually increasing as your jaw strength improves. Avoid excessive force to prevent strain.

Why It Works: Strengthens the jaw and facial muscles, improving overall punch resistance.

If you're serious about boxing, neck training is not optional—it's a necessity. A well-trained neck can be the difference between staying in the fight or staying on the canvas.

Train your neck. Build your chin. Step into the ring knowing you can take anything thrown at you.

True Champs Eat Body Shots

Taking punches to the body can be a brutal experience, but developing resistance to body shots is required for any serious boxer. While core exercises can help strengthen the muscles, the only true way to adapt to body shots is through gradual and controlled exposure to impact. This chapter will explore different methods to build up your body shot resistance and highlight how some of the sport's greatest fighters have developed their ability to take body shots.

The Importance of Body Shot Resistance

Body shots can end fights instantly. A well-placed punch to the liver or solar plexus has dropped even the toughest warriors. To minimize this risk, fighters must develop the ability to absorb and recover from these blows.

Muscle strength helps, but real body shot resistance is built through proper breathing, reflexive bracing, and repeated exposure to impact.

Methods to Build Body Shot Resistance

Medicine Ball Drops: Have a partner lightly throw or drop a medicine ball onto your stomach. As your tolerance builds, gradually increase the weight of the ball and the intensity of the drops. This mimics the impact of body punches and conditions your muscles to handle real hits.

Controlled Body Punches: During training, have a partner throw measured, controlled punches to your stomach and sides. Start light and progressively increase the force. This trains your body and mind to withstand real fight conditions.

Stick Drills: This drill involves a partner hitting your core and arms with a stick. It conditions the body to handle repeated impacts and increases pain tolerance.

Core Exercises for Boxers

In addition to impact conditioning, a strong core helps you absorb punches better without breaking down or fatiguing as quickly.

For detailed information on strengthening the core, refer to the Core Stability chapter.

How the Greats Conditioned Themselves for Body Shots

Sugar Ray Robinson: One of the greatest boxers of all time, Sugar Ray Robinson, incorporated medicine ball throws into his training. Videos show his trainer crashing a medicine ball into his stomach, helping him develop incredible resistance to body shots.

Manny Pacquiao: Renowned for his toughness, Manny Pacquiao used stick drills to build remarkable body shot resistance. By enduring hits around his core and arms with a stick, Pacquiao conditioned his body to withstand repeated impacts and pain, contributing to his ability to take powerful shots and continue fighting effectively.

Timothy Bradley: Bradley is another example of a fighter with outstanding body shot resistance. His rigorous training regimen included various core-strengthening and body-conditioning exercises that helped him absorb and recover from punishing body blows throughout his career.

Several other renowned boxers have similarly focused on body shot resistance. Techniques such as using medicine balls and controlled body punches are staples in the training routines of many champions, allowing them to endure and recover from body shots that might incapacitate less conditioned fighters.

Gradual Exposure and Consistency

Building resistance to body shots requires a gradual process. Abruptly increasing the intensity of impacts can lead to injury, so it's important to start slowly and progressively increase the force and volume of impacts.

Just like punch resistance for the head, body shot conditioning requires consistency. Done regularly, this training hardens your body to pressure and makes you much harder to break down.

Stretching: Unlocking Speed, Fluidity, Power, and Endurance

Fighters instinctively know that feeling tight and restricted is the enemy of performance. To stay fast, fluid, and explosive, you need mobility that allows for seamless movement and split-second reactions.

If you're not stretching, you're limiting your potential. Simple as that. Stretching is not only about avoiding injury, but also about unlocking physical attributes that would otherwise be trapped. Think of it as trapped energy—the more relaxed and fluid your muscles are, the more blood can flow throughout your body, indirectly enhancing endurance, speed, and power.

Just look at Dmitry Bivol. Known for his relaxed, fluid style, Bivol's flexibility and loose, controlled movement allow him to strike with precision while keeping a high punch output without fading. His ability to stay mobile and efficient deep into fights suggests the benefits of flexibility and mobility, which allow fighters to move freely without excess energy expenditure. Gennady "GGG" Golovkin was a strong proponent of stretching, reportedly incorporating multiple stretching sessions throughout the day; before his morning run, before gym training, and after workouts. His focus on flexibility contributed to his ability to stay loose, balanced, and maintain power deep into fights.

Dynamic Stretching: Prepping for Action

Dynamic stretching gets your body warmed up, loosening muscles and joints while preparing you for the demands of training. It improves your range of motion, primes your body for explosive movements, and ensures you stay light on your feet. This type of stretching helps you stay agile, powerful, and ready for high-intensity movements in the ring.

When to Do Dynamic Stretching:

Pre-Workout: Use dynamic stretches before training or sparring to prepare muscles for action.

Before Intense Drills: Perform these stretches to ensure your body is primed for quick, high-impact movements.

If your body feels extra tight before training, you can briefly hold isolated stretches for about 10–15 seconds to loosen stubborn areas, then transition into dynamic movements. Sometimes, tight muscles need priming before they're ready to move explosively.

Examples of Dynamic Stretches:

Leg Swings: Stand on one leg, swing the opposite leg forward and backward for 10 to 12 swings per leg. Then swing it side to side across your body for another 10 to 12 swings. This opens up the hips, loosens the hamstrings, and activates the lower body for movement.

High Knees: Run in place, bringing your knees up toward your chest for 20 to 30 seconds.

Arm Circles: Make large forward and backward circles with your arms for 20 to 30 seconds.

Broomstick Rotations: Hold a stick or dowel across your shoulders behind your head, and rotate your torso side to side for 20 to 30 seconds. This warms up the spine, shoulders, and core—great for prepping rotational movements like punches and slips.

Lunges with a Twist: Step forward into a lunge, twist your torso, and return to the starting position. Perform 8–10 reps per side.

Static Stretching: Recovery and Flexibility

After the grind of training, static stretching (where you hold a stretch without moving for 10 to 30 seconds plus) helps your muscles cool down, reduces soreness, and increases flexibility. Holding these stretches allows your muscles to fully relax, improving range of motion and helping you recover faster. Better flexibility means your muscles move with less tension and use less energy, which indirectly boosts endurance and stamina.

When to Do Static Stretching

Post-Workout: After training, use static stretches to cool down and keep your muscles loose.

Recovery Days: Stretch on off days to prevent stiffness and maintain mobility.

Examples of Static Stretches:

Hamstring Stretch: Sit with one leg extended and the other bent, and reach toward the toes of the extended leg to stretch your hamstrings, keeping your legs flexible for better movement and balance.

Quadriceps Stretch: Stand on one leg and pull the opposite foot toward your glutes, keeping your knees together and hips pushed slightly forward to stretch the front of your thigh. This helps maintain flexibility in the quadriceps, reducing tightness that can restrict movement and footwork.

Hip Flexor Stretch: Kneel on one knee with the other foot in front, gently push your hips forward to stretch your hip flexors, keeping your hips loose for fluid footwork.

Calf Stretch: Stand with one leg forward and the other extended back, press the heel of the back foot into the ground to stretch your calves, helping you stay light on your feet.

Chest (Pec) Stretch: Stand in a doorway, place both hands on the frame at shoulder height, and step forward slightly to open up the chest.

Shoulder Stretch: Bring one arm across your chest and use the opposite hand to pull it closer, loosening your shoulders and preventing restrictions during punches.

Triceps Stretch: Reach one arm overhead and bend the elbow, using the opposite hand to press it further down the back, improving flexibility for better punching extension.

The Importance of Blood Flow in Boxing Performance

Stretching plays a major role in increasing blood flow, which directly enhances your performance in the ring. Here's how improved circulation helps:

Improved Oxygen Delivery: Stretching boosts blood flow, bringing oxygen-rich blood to your muscles. This oxygen fuels your muscles and allows them to produce energy more efficiently, helping you perform longer without tiring, thus improving endurance.

Nutrient Transport: Better circulation delivers essential nutrients like glucose, fueling your muscles for powerful movements and aiding in faster recovery. This means your muscles stay fresh longer, reducing the drop in output as rounds progress.

Faster Waste Removal: Stretching helps increase circulation, clearing out metabolic waste like lactic acid, which builds up during intense exercise. This reduces soreness and speeds recovery, ensuring you get back to training without feeling sluggish.

Mobility Work: Ensuring Smooth Movement

Mobility work—things like foam rolling, dynamic stretches, and even yoga—keeps your body moving the way it's supposed to. It improves how your muscles and joints function, lowers your risk of injury, and helps you stay sharp in the ring. Foam rolling loosens up tight spots, making your movement smoother, while yoga boosts flexibility and keeps your mind dialed in. Both help you recover faster and keep your body running at its best.

Foam Rolling: Roll targeted areas of your body to loosen tight muscles and improve mobility. Focus on high-tension areas such as the calves, quads, hamstrings, and lower back, as these directly affect footwork and overall movement.

Hip Openers: Perform Lunging Hip Flexor Stretches by stepping one foot forward into a lunge, keeping the back leg extended and hips square. Sink into the stretch with an upright torso. Hold for 30 seconds on each side. This helps improve footwork mobility, reduces energy leaks during punches, and enhances lateral explosiveness.

Third World Squat: With feet shoulder-width apart and toes slightly turned out, lower your hips into a deep squat while keeping your heels flat on the ground. Hold for 30 seconds to 2 minutes. This boosts ankle, knee, and hip mobility, helping you stay grounded and balanced during evasive movement or close-range exchanges.

Yoga: Practice poses that develop flexibility, balance, and mental clarity.

- *Cat-Cow Stretch*: On hands and knees, inhale while arching your back (Cow), exhale while rounding it (Cat). Repeat for 30–60 seconds to improve spinal mobility and rotational ability for punches and slips.

- *Warrior's Pose*: From a standing lunge, turn your back foot out, raise arms overhead, and bend the front knee. Builds lower-body strength and base stability.

- *Tree Pose*: Stand tall, place one foot on the opposite inner thigh or calf, and balance with palms together in front of the chest. Sharpens focus and balance.

- *Downward Dog*: From hands and knees, lift your hips up and back to form an inverted V. Stretches the posterior chain and enhances full-body mobility.

Round 7: Recovery & Nutrition

Chapter 37
Fueling the Fighter: The Importance of Food Quality and Nutrition

"I don't eat to die, I eat to live." [50]
—Bernard Hopkins

As a fighter striving for greatness, your success depends on more than just training and technique; it also relies on what you put into your body. Some athletes focus solely on counting calories, believing that eating less than they burn is the key to making weight. Others ignore food quality completely and just focus on cutting pounds as the fight gets closer. However, the caliber of your diet matters far more than simply reducing intake.

Think of your body like a high-performance car. Just as a car needs premium fuel to run efficiently and last longer, your body thrives on high-quality food. If you fuel a car with cheap, low-grade gasoline, it might run for a while, but eventually, its performance will drop, and it won't last as long. The same applies to your body; feeding it processed, nutrient-poor foods may keep you going temporarily, but over time, your energy, recovery, and overall performance will suffer.

Do you want to eat unhealthy foods because they "taste good" while gasping for air in the ring as your opponent is teeing off on you? Or do you want to eat clean foods so you can perform at your full ability?

To be at your best, you need to fuel your body with the right foods.

---

[50] Hopkins, Bernard. Quoted in an interview with *Men's Health*, February 2014. The former middleweight and light heavyweight champion was discussing his strict nutrition regimen and longevity in the sport.

The Pitfalls of Counting Calories

While consuming fewer calories than you burn can lead to weight loss, it neglects the importance of proper nutrition. Not all calories are equal. Your body needs quality fuel to perform at its best, not just a specific number of calories. Fast food, sugary snacks, and refined carbs may be satisfying in the moment, but they offer no value for performance.

Clean, nutrient-dense foods not only fuel your body but also naturally support weight loss.

When your body gets the nutrients it needs, digestion improves, bloating decreases, and metabolism stays steady—eliminating the need for extreme calorie cutting.

A 2019 study by the National Institutes of Health (NIH) showed that people who ate a diet heavy in processed foods gained more weight compared to those who focused on natural, whole foods, even when calorie intake was the same. The takeaway: prioritize nutrient-rich, whole foods for better results.

The Power of Nutrient-Dense Foods

Whole, unprocessed foods—such as fruits, vegetables, lean proteins, and whole grains—are packed with essential vitamins, minerals, and fiber without adding empty calories. These nutrients are crucial for muscle growth, recovery, immune strength, and mental clarity.

Choosing whole grains over sugary treats, lean cuts of meat over fatty ones, and healthy fats like nuts and avocado instead of trans fats will improve your overall performance and health. Including a variety of colorful fruits and vegetables makes sure your body gets key nutrients like vitamin D for bone strength and iron for oxygen transport.

The Impact of Food Quality on Digestion and Absorption

The type of food you eat also affects how well your body processes and absorbs nutrients. Whole, natural foods are generally easier for your body to digest, leading to better nutrient absorption. Processed foods can trigger inflammation, weaken digestion, and limit nutrient absorption. This drains your energy and slows recovery. Many contain additives and preservatives that worsen the issue.

Fueling Your Body for Boxing Greatness

To succeed in the ring, your nutrition plan should focus on providing the right nutrients to optimize performance, speed up recovery, and maintain overall health. Bernard Hopkins is a perfect example of this mindset. He famously fought at a world-class level into his late 40s—not because of some secret supplement, but because of relentless discipline with how he treated his body. Hopkins saw food not as instant gratification, but as fuel for greatness. That level of commitment extended his prime long after most fighters had faded. Prioritize natural, nutrient-dense foods while minimizing processed options that offer little value.

Structure your meals around lean proteins, complex carbohydrates, and healthy fats to support muscle development, sustain energy, and boost brain function. Including a variety of fruits and vegetables ensures your body gets the full range of vitamins and minerals it needs. Don't forget hydration—it's one of the most important and most overlooked parts of a fighter's performance. Your body runs on water just as much as food.

After high-intensity workouts, you should replenish your glycogen stores (the energy reserves your muscles rely on during exercise) by consuming fast-digesting carbohydrates, such as fruits, white rice, or plain potatoes, alongside a source of protein. This helps speed up recovery and prepares your body for the next training session.

General Amount of Protein, Carbs, and Fats

For fighters, getting the right balance of protein, carbohydrates, and fats is important to reach your best performance and recover properly. Here's a simple guide for daily intake based on your weight:

Protein: Aim for 0.7 to 1.1 grams per pound of body weight (1.6 to 2.4 grams per kilogram).

Protein helps build and repair muscles.

Carbohydrates: Aim for 1.5 to 3.2 grams per pound of body weight (3.5 to 7 grams per kilogram).

Carbs give you energy for training and help refill your energy stores.

Fats: Aim for 0.2 to 0.7 grams of fat per pound of body weight (or 0.5 to 1.5 grams per kilogram).

Healthy fats provide long-lasting energy and support overall health.

These ranges apply to training and performance phases. During a weight cut, adjustments may be necessary, but always prioritize recovery and energy.

The Building Blocks of a Fighter's Diet

Here are examples of each nutrient type to incorporate into your meal planning:

Complex Carbohydrates: Quinoa, oats, sweet potatoes, lentils, chickpeas, black beans, and high-quality whole grain breads like Ezekiel or traditional sourdough.

(**Note:** While white rice and plain potatoes aren't complex carbs, they are excellent for fast glycogen replenishment post-training.)

Lean Proteins: Chicken breast, turkey, salmon, lean ground beef, eggs, Greek yogurt, cottage cheese, bone broth protein, and optional plant-based protein powders if tolerated.

(**Note:** On recovery days, a high-quality ribeye steak can be a great way to refuel after hard sparring or strength sessions, it's rich in nutrients and satisfying. But limit red meat intake overall, as fattier cuts like ribeye take longer to digest and may not sit well before intense training.)

Healthy Fats: Avocado, almonds, chia seeds, flaxseeds, olive oil, macadamia nuts, and walnuts.

(**Note:** Coconut oil can also be used in moderation, its medium-chain fats digest quickly and can provide a fast energy source, especially during training camps or cutting phases.)

Fruits (Fast-Acting Carbs): Bananas, berries, oranges, apples, grapes, dates, and pineapple. (Great for quick energy and replenishing glycogen stores after intense workouts.)

Vegetables: Broccoli, spinach, kale, bell peppers, Brussels sprouts, cauliflower, and sweet potatoes. (Rich in vitamins, minerals, and fiber to support overall health and performance.)

Foods to Avoid

Just as important as knowing what to eat is knowing what to avoid. Fighters should steer clear of foods that sabotage energy, slow recovery, and cause inflammation. These include:

• Sugary drinks like soda, sweetened iced tea, and energy drinks.

• Fast food (burgers, fries, fried chicken, etc.).

• Refined sugars and processed snacks (candy bars, pastries, cookies, and sugary cereals).

• Processed meats (hot dogs, sausages, deli meats with preservatives).

• Trans fats and highly processed oils (hydrogenated oils, margarine, canola, soybean, corn, and other industrial seed oils commonly found in packaged snacks and baked goods).

• Alcohol (it dehydrates you, impairs recovery, and affects sleep quality).

• Artificial sweeteners and chemical-filled foods with long ingredient lists you can't pronounce.

If you can't pronounce it or it has a long list of ingredients, it probably doesn't belong in a fighter's diet.

These foods can lead to sluggishness, poor digestion, brain fog, and even increased risk of injury due to chronic inflammation.

What you eat shows up in how you train, how you recover, and how you perform. There's no escaping it. You either fuel like a fighter or gas out and regret it.

Do you have to be perfect 24/7?

No. If you have a craving, go for it. Just don't make it a habit. And here's the truth, there are ways to make healthy food taste incredible, even desserts. You just have to expand your mindset, get creative, and stay conscious of what you're putting in your body. That kind of awareness is what leads to long-term sustainability.

Example Meals

For those looking for structure, here are some easy-to-follow meal plans:

Daily Menu 1

- Breakfast: Overnight oats with mixed berries, chia seeds, and a boiled egg.

- Snack: Greek yogurt with sliced almonds and a drizzle of honey.

- Lunch: Grilled chicken with quinoa, roasted sweet potato, and steamed broccoli.

- Post-Workout Snack: Hard-boiled eggs with a small handful of almonds. (Note: To replenish glycogen, consider adding a carbohydrate source like a banana or rice cakes.)

- Dinner: Baked salmon with roasted asparagus and steamed lentils. *(Provides omega-3s, lean protein, and slow-digesting carbs for muscle recovery.)*

Daily Menu 2

- Breakfast: Spinach and feta omelet with whole-grain toast and avocado slices.

- Snack: Cottage cheese with pineapple and a sprinkle of cinnamon.

- Lunch: Turkey and avocado wrap in a whole-wheat tortilla with lettuce and tomato.

- Post-Workout Snack: Scrambled eggs with toast and a side of fruit. (Alternatively, you can opt for a protein shake with added fruit for both protein and carbs to aid recovery.)

- Dinner: Grilled steak with sautéed spinach and mashed sweet potatoes. *(Great for iron intake, muscle repair, and glycogen replenishment.)*

Basic Snack Ideas

Here are some quick and simple snack options to help fuel your training:

- Fruit with a handful of nuts.

- Rice cakes with almond butter.

- Greek yogurt with honey.

- Cottage cheese with fruit.

- Hard-boiled eggs.

How Your Body Uses Energy During Exercise

Your body uses different energy sources: carbohydrates, proteins, and fats, depending on how hard you're working. The type of fuel your body burns changes based on the intensity of your exercise. Here's a breakdown of how your body shifts between these energy sources:

Energy Use Based on Exercise Intensity

High Intensity (8-10):

When you're going all out—hard sparring, explosive pad work, or intense bag drills—your body runs almost entirely on carbohydrates.

If your glycogen stores are low, your body might start breaking down muscle protein. That's something you absolutely want to avoid.

Fat isn't used much during this stage, but it kicks in during recovery once the heart rate drops.

Moderate Intensity (4-7):

At this level, think steady bag work or light sparring, your body uses a mix of carbs and fat.

Fat starts to play a bigger role, but carbs still fuel most movements. Protein stays mostly untouched unless your carb intake is too low.

Low Intensity (1-3):

When the pace is slow (light jogging, walking, mobility drills, etc) your body burns mostly fat.

At this level, fat is the primary fuel, with just a little help from carbs and almost no protein unless you're fasting or underfed.

Why This Matters for Fighters

Understanding how your body uses energy at different intensities helps you plan meals for better performance and endurance.

For high-intensity sessions (sparring, explosive pad work), eat more carbs beforehand to ensure your muscles have the fuel they need.

For moderate-intensity training (steady bag work, drills), balance carbs and fats for sustained energy.

For low-intensity sessions or rest days, focus on healthy fats for long-lasting fuel.

How to Measure Intensity:

Intensity is commonly measured using perceived exertion, how hard you feel you're working. One simple way to gauge it is by using a 0-10 scale:

- 0 = Resting (no effort at all).
- 10 = Maximum effort (as hard as you can possibly go).
- Moderate intensity (4-7) should feel like steady effort, while high intensity (8-10) should push you close to your limit.

Tailoring Your Fuel for Performance

This is a general guide. Individual needs vary, especially for fighters in different weight classes or training schedules.

For precise meal planning, consulting a sports nutritionist is best. They can tailor a diet based on your fight camp schedule, weight cut, and recovery needs.

Chapter 38
Performance: Enhancing Supplements for the Boxer

Becoming the best version of yourself as a fighter means maximizing every part of your training, recovery, and performance. While a strong diet, consistent training, and plenty of rest lay the groundwork, the right supplements can help take your results up a notch. Before adding any supplements to your regimen, consult a doctor or sports nutritionist to make sure they're appropriate and safe for your body. This chapter covers some of the most effective, science-backed supplements to boost endurance, speed up recovery, and improve performance in the ring.

The Role of Supplements

Supplements are meant to complement, not replace, a solid nutrition plan. They help fill in nutritional gaps and offer targeted benefits when paired with proper training and recovery routines.

Key Supplements for Boxers

Creatine Monohydrate

Creatine is one of the most researched and effective supplements for enhancing athletic performance.

What it does: Helps increase muscle mass, boosts strength, and speeds up recovery after intense workouts.

How much to take: 3-5 grams daily, typically in powder or capsule form.

New research: Higher daily doses have also been linked to cognitive benefits, such as improved mental clarity and reduced fatigue — potentially giving fighters an edge in focus and decision-making during training and competition.[51]

Beta-Alanine

This amino acid helps buffer acid buildup in your muscles during high-intensity exercise, allowing you to push through tough workouts.

What it does: Improves endurance, increases strength, and helps you maintain performance during intense sessions.

How much to take: 2-5 grams per day, usually taken as a powder or capsule.

Note: Beta-alanine often causes a tingling sensation on the face and ears, known as *The Beta-Alanine Tingle*. This is harmless and typically wears off after a short time.

Caffeine

Caffeine is a powerful tool for improving focus and endurance, but it should be used carefully.

What it does: Increases alertness, boosts endurance, and enhances performance.

How much to take: 3-6 mg per kg of body weight, 30-60 minutes before training. *(For reference, this is about one to two cups of drip coffee per 150 lbs (68 kg) of body weight.)*

---

[51] University of Kansas Medical Center, "Creatine shows potential to boost cognition in Alzheimer's patients," *KU Medical Center News*, June 4, 2025.

Note: Keep an eye on caffeine intake—too much can cause jitteriness, spike cortisol, or overexcite the nervous system. Caffeine can stay in your system for eight or more hours depending on your metabolism and tolerance, so consuming it too late in the day may interfere with sleep quality and recovery. The highest-level approach is to rely on your own natural energy and avoid caffeine altogether. If you choose to use it, treat it like a performance-day edge, used sparingly and with purpose, because over time it can dull your real energy and create dependency.

Beetroot Powder and Whole Beets

Beetroot is loaded with nitrates that increase nitric oxide production in your body, improving blood flow and oxygen efficiency. Beetroot powder is a convenient option, but whole beets work well too.

What it does: Boosts endurance, improves cardiovascular performance, and enhances muscle efficiency.

How much to take: 3-6 grams of beetroot powder (or two to three medium-sized beets) two to three hours before training.

Protein *Supplements*

While whole foods are always the best source of protein, supplements can help you hit your daily protein needs, especially when you're training hard.

What it does: Aids muscle recovery, supports muscle growth, and provides an easy source of high-quality protein.

How much to take: 20-40 grams post-workout or whenever needed to meet daily protein goals.

Essential Amino Acids (EAAs)

These are the building blocks of protein, and since your body can't produce them on its own, you need to get them through food or supplements.

What it does: Promotes muscle protein synthesis, speeds up recovery, and helps reduce muscle soreness.
How much to take: 5-10 grams before, during, or after exercise.

Fish Oil (*Omega*-3 Fatty Acids)

Omega-3s in fish oil help reduce inflammation and improve recovery, making them a valuable tool for any boxer.

What it does: Reduces inflammation, supports joint health, aids in recovery, and benefits your cardiovascular system.
How much to take: 1-3 grams of combined EPA and DHA per day.

Electrolytes (Potassium, Magnesium, Sodium)

Intense training and heavy sweating can cause your body to lose important electrolytes, especially potassium and magnesium. These are essential for muscle function, hydration, and preventing cramps. Replenishing electrolytes through food and supplements can help you stay balanced and energized, especially after tough training sessions.

What they do: Help maintain hydration, keep your muscles working properly, prevent cramps, and support energy levels during long or intense training.

How much to take per mineral

Potassium: Athletes need more potassium than the average person, but getting enough from food alone can be difficult. While daily recommendations suggest around 4,000-4,700 mg, that doesn't mean you need to eat 10 bananas a day! Electrolyte supplements are a simple way to make sure you're getting enough, especially after a heavy sweat session. You can also boost your intake with potassium-rich foods like avocados, spinach, sweet potatoes, and coconut water.

Magnesium (Magnesium Glycinate): Aim for around 200–400 mg per day. Magnesium is crucial for muscle relaxation, recovery, and preventing cramps. Magnesium glycinate, in particular, is one of the most absorbable and gentle forms , making it especially good for athletes. It also supports your central nervous system, improves sleep, and speeds up recovery after intense training. Foods like leafy greens, nuts, and seeds also contain magnesium, but many athletes benefit from supplementing this specific form.

Sodium: Because sodium is lost heavily in sweat, make sure to replace it, especially during or after long, intense workouts. Electrolyte drinks or adding a pinch of salt to your food can help replenish sodium levels. Depending on your training and sweat levels, you may need 500-2,300 mg of sodium per day.

Additional Supplements Worth Considering

L-Citrulline and L-Arginine

These amino acids help increase nitric oxide production, improving blood flow and endurance during training. Watermelon is a natural source of citrulline, making it a great food to include for this effect.

What it does: Boosts nitric oxide, enhances blood flow, and improves endurance and muscle performance.

How much to take: 6-8 grams of L-citrulline or L-arginine per day, or enjoy a couple of large slices of watermelon before training.

Glutamine

Glutamine is an amino acid that supports immune health and may aid in muscle recovery, especially during intense training periods.

What it does: May help reduce muscle soreness and support immune function during heavy training cycles.

How much to take: 5-10 grams per day.

Note: If you're already getting enough protein from your diet, the additional benefits from glutamine may be limited.

Cordyceps Mushrooms

What it does: May improve oxygen use energy production, and reduce fatigue. Some users also report improved mental clarity due to better endurance and stress resilience.

How much to take: 1-3 grams per day, typically in extract or capsule form.

Rhodiola Rosea

What it does: Helps the body handle physical and mental stress, potentially boosting endurance.

How much to take: 200-600 mg per day, ideally standardized to 3% rosavins and 1% salidroside.

Ashwagandha

What it does: A powerful adaptogen known to help the body manage stress, improve strength, and support stamina and recovery.

How much to take: 300–600 mg per day, usually standardized to 5% withanolides (the active compounds that give ashwagandha its stress-relief and performance-boosting effects).

Taurine

What it does: Supports muscle function and endurance, which is beneficial for boxers.

How much to take: 1-3 grams per day, taken pre-workout or throughout the day.

Vitamin D3 + K2

What it does: Supports bone health, immune function, and hormone balance, which is especially important for athletes training indoors or in areas with limited sunlight.

How much to take: 2,000-5,000 IU of Vitamin D3 with 100-200 mcg of Vitamin K2 per day.

Collagen (with Vitamin C)

What it does: Aids in tendon, ligament, and joint health, especially useful for boxers dealing with wear and tear on hands, shoulders, and knees. Taking it with vitamin C enhances collagen synthesis.

How much to take: 10-15 grams of collagen with 50-100 mg of vitamin C per day, ideally one hour before training or as part of your daily routine.

Curcumin (Turmeric Extract)

What it does: Potent anti-inflammatory compound that supports joint health and recovery, helping reduce soreness and inflammation after intense sessions.

How much to take: 500-1,000 mg per day, preferably with black pepper extract to enhance absorption.

Supplements: A Tool, Not a Shortcut

Supplements can support training and recovery, but they are not a replacement for hard work, a balanced diet, and rest. Before adding new supplements into your regimen, consult a healthcare provider or sports nutritionist to ensure they fit your needs and are safe to use.

Make sure you're purchasing from trusted brands to avoid unwanted or banned substances. Stay informed about your sport's regulations, some supplements may be restricted in competition, so always check with your governing body.

Keep in mind, this list isn't meant to be all-encompassing. These are simply some of the most proven and practical supplements for boxing performance, a starting point for you to explore. Every fighter is unique, so do your own research, and listen to your body. Consider this chapter your doorway into the world of performance nutrition. Where you go from here is up to you.

Quick-Reference Cheat Sheet: Key Supplements for Boxers

Supplement	Benefit	Recommended Dose
Creatine Monohydrate	Strength, power, recovery	3–5 g per day
Beta-Alanine	Endurance, buffers acid buildup	2–5 g per day
Caffeine	Alertness, focus, endurance	3–6 mg per kg of bodyweight. 30–60 min pre-workout — use sparingly; can dull natural energy over time
Beetroot Powder	Blood flow, stamina	3–6 g powder (2–3 hrs pre-training)
Protein (Bone broth or Vegan)	Muscle recovery and growth	20–40 g post-workout
Essential Amino Acids (EAAs)	Muscle protein synthesis	5–10 g pre-/intra-/ post-workout
Fish Oil (EPA + DHA)	Recovery, joint health, anti-inflammatory	1–3 g per day
Potassium	Muscle function, hydration	Get 4,000–4,700 mg daily (food + supplements)
Magnesium Glycinate	Muscle relaxation, recovery, CNS support	200–400 mg per day
Sodium	Hydration, muscle contraction	500–2,300 mg per day (as needed)

Supplement	Benefit	Recommended Dose
L-Citrulline/ L-Arginine	Blood flow, endurance	6–8 g pre-training
Glutamine	Immune support, recovery	5–10 g per day
Cordyceps Mushrooms	Energy, oxygen use	1–3 g per day
Rhodiola Rosea	Stress resilience, endurance	200–600 mg per day
Ashwagandha	Stress management, stamina, recovery	300–600 mg per day
Taurine	Muscle endurance	1–3 g per day
Vitamin D3 + K2	Bone health, immune function	2,000–5,000 IU D3 + 100–200 mcg K2 per day
Collagen + Vitamin C	Tendon & joint support	10–15 g collagen + 50–100 mg vit C per day
Curcumin	Anti-inflammatory, joint health	500–1,000 mg per day (with black pepper extract)

In the end, supplements are just tools to help maximize the work you're already putting in. Your dedication, skill, and sweat will always be the real key to success in the ring. Supplements? They're just there to help you get the most out of your efforts.

Chapter 39
The Infamous Weight Cut: Art and Science

As a fighter, achieving the right weight class can be just as important as training and technique. Striking a balance between cutting weight (or not) and maintaining peak performance is key to your success in the ring.

The goal? To fight in the lowest possible weight class without sacrificing performance, giving you a potential size and strength advantage over your opponent.

Don't get me wrong: size can definitely be an advantage if the fighter hasn't been drained by an aggressive weight cut. There are weight classes for a reason, but size alone isn't an advantage. Strength, endurance, and skill are what truly matter. Whether you're an amateur going three fast-paced rounds on the same day as weigh-ins, a pro fighting a four-rounder, or competing at the highest level in a 12-round championship bout, entering the ring depleted can hurt your performance.

In combat sports, endurance is critical across all disciplines. While MMA incorporates grappling opportunities that shift energy demands to different muscle groups or systems, boxing's constant movement and striking output require sustained energy while remaining on your feet. The risks of cutting too much weight are magnified for amateur boxers, who have less recovery time (same day weigh-ins), and for longer professional fights, where stamina and endurance are necessary. Amateurs typically weigh in on the morning of the fight itself, while professionals usually weigh in at least 24 hours before their bout, allowing them more time to recover.

That said, it's easier to get away with the effects of a hard weight cut in a 4-, 6-, or even 8-round fight, especially if the opponent isn't applying relentless pressure. But the deeper the rounds go, and the higher the caliber of fighter you're facing, the more those hidden consequences start to surface. What felt manageable early on becomes a liability when fatigue creeps in, reactions slow, and the sharpness fades. You can't fake energy or grit when you're sapped of strength. Over the championship distance, the cost of a tough weight cut usually gets exposed.

Cutting a manageable amount of weight to compete in the right class can give you an edge if done safely. But the moment the cut crosses into extreme territory, that edge turns into vulnerability, your timing, endurance, and sharpness all take a hit.

The fighters who cut significant weight and still perform are exceptions, not the rule. Their success is a mix of genetic factors, recovery strategies, and elite preparation. Access to advanced sports science, experienced nutritionists, and recovery protocols can make or break a cut, enabling some fighters to perform well despite the strain of significant weight loss. Even so, they often do so at less than optimal capacity, regardless of whether they win. While it's possible, the hidden toll makes it a dangerous approach for most fighters. This is why cutting safely is so critical to performing at your peak in the ring.

Having a tough weight cut can work if you're significantly better than your opponent. But it's a gamble, and not recommended to pursue an overzealous cut just for the size advantage.

There are times where boxers have used extreme methods, like severe calorie restriction, going without food or water, and spitting in a cup for hours to shed pounds rapidly. While these techniques can help a fighter make weight, they often leave the body running on fumes, impacting energy levels, endurance, and performance in the ring. Today, with advances in sports science, there are safer, more effective approaches that prioritize both health and performance.

The Risks of Rapid Weight Loss

Cutting weight too quickly, especially through dehydration, can severely affect your performance. Research has shown that losing as little as 3% of your body weight through dehydration can reduce your performance by up to 30%, decreasing your energy, power, and mental sharpness. In a sport where split-second decisions and reactions can mean the difference between victory and defeat, this drop in performance can be catastrophic.

Boxing is not limited to size. Strength, speed, endurance, and skills matter most. Many successful fighters have understood that entering the ring at their peak, rather than drained from a brutal weight cut, is far more important than squeezing into a lower weight class. As Oleksandr Usyk put it, *"Size doesn't matter. If only size mattered then the elephant would be the king of the jungle."*

Gradual Weight Loss: The Safe Approach

The best way to cut weight is gradually, through a smart diet and exercise plan. Gradual weight loss keeps you hydrated and ensures your body stays balanced. Aim to spar as close to your target weight as possible during training camp to avoid last-minute drastic cuts.

If you're unsure of the best weight to fight at, it's often close to your natural weight—the weight where you feel strong, fast, and energized. You can find your natural weight through the process of eating clean and training hard. By focusing on building lean muscle and losing fat, your body will naturally settle into the weight that's ideal for your performance.

For example, when I was fighting at 141 pounds as an amateur for a big tournament, I spent most of the camp in a serious calorie deficit just to make weight. After an exhausting 12-mile run, I only lost half a pound. My body was telling me it had nothing left to give, so I decided it was time to move up. Some people thought I was too small for the next weight class up at 152 pounds and warned me I'd be undersized against naturally bigger, stronger guys. But I decided to listen to my body, not the doubters. Moving up paid off immediately. My first fight at 152 was a first-round TKO. My power, speed, and energy were at their peak and my performances kept improving. That choice to fight closer to my natural weight let me truly shine and proved that feeling strong and healthy is far more important than squeezing into a weight class just because you can.

Your natural body type also plays a major role in how you respond to a weight cut. Fighters with leaner, ectomorph builds often have less body fat and glycogen (carbohydrates) to lose, making extreme cuts riskier and more likely to result in strength or endurance loss. Mesomorphs, naturally muscular athletes, may tolerate moderate cuts better, maintaining power and energy if recovery is done right. Endomorphs, who tend to carry more mass or fat, might cut larger amounts but are also more vulnerable to fatigue, sluggishness, or water retention issues if the cut is mismanaged. Knowing your body type and adjusting your strategy accordingly can make the difference between a safe cut and one that drains your performance.

The 10-Day Weight Cut Plan

(Note: This plan is geared toward experienced fighters)

If you choose to cut weight, doing it properly is the key. Here's a framework to help you manage it safely and effectively.

While most of your weight loss should happen gradually throughout training camp, the final 10 days before the weigh-in are critical for fine-tuning your weight and ensuring peak performance.

This plan is geared toward professional fighters with experience in managing weight cuts. Below is a step-by-step guide to help you through this process, assuming your weigh-ins are on a Friday.

It's important to note that this plan is just an example and should be tailored to individual needs. Consulting a nutritionist or healthcare professional is advised to create a safe, personalized approach.

10 Days Before Weigh-in:

- Start drinking more water, around two gallons per day. This "water loading" phase triggers your body's flushing mechanisms, making it easier to shed water weight later in the cut.

7 Days Before Weigh-in:

- Gradually reduce portion sizes and eliminate processed foods, sugars, and excess carbohydrates from your diet.

- Along with reducing portion sizes, focus on nutrient-dense, light foods that help you feel satisfied without weighing you down. Salads with lean protein, bone broth-based soups, and seafood are great options, they provide essential nutrients, support digestion, and promote a lighter, leaner feel leading into fight week.

- Continue high water intake to maintain hydration and help with water flushing.

- Begin to reduce sodium intake moderately, focusing on natural, minimally salted foods to support electrolyte balance. This moderate reduction prepares your body to release water weight.

5 Days Before Weigh-in:

- Further reduce salt intake to minimize water retention while keeping your high-water routine.

- Use green tea or black coffee with coconut oil to support fat loss. If you choose a caffeinated option, keep the dose minimal and treat it as a short-term tool during the cut, not a daily habit, to avoid dulling your natural energy or creating dependency.

- Keep sodium at minimal levels rather than fully eliminating it, as small amounts are essential for muscle contraction and can prevent cramping.

"Fight Week" (Three Days Before Weigh-in):

- Gradually reduce water intake, but continue drinking small amounts with lemon juice to maintain alkalinity.

- Begin using natural diuretics like 1500mg of dandelion root and 1500mg of uva ursi, three times a day, to help release water.[52]

- Use very minimal sodium and remove carbohydrates from your diet completely to help your body release water more easily.

- Limit potassium at this stage, as it can cause water retention, but keep a small amount as needed for muscle function.

2 Days Before Weigh-in:

- Eat small, lean protein meals with minimal sodium every three hours.

- Continue using natural diuretics.

1 Day Before Weigh-in:

- Take 1800 mg of senna at night to assist with bowel movements, helping to shed the last bit of weight. Be cautious, as overuse can lead to dehydration or electrolyte imbalances.

- Reduce water intake, but drink small sips of ice-cold water when needed.

- If necessary, use a sauna suit or steam room to shed the final pounds, but monitor your hydration carefully to avoid excessive water loss.

- Another method that can help shed water weight is hot bath soaks. However, this method strips your body of essential minerals like sodium, potassium, and magnesium, which are crucial for performance. Use this technique cautiously, as it can leave you feeling depleted.

---

[52] Lockhart, George. *Nutrition and Weight Cutting Principles for Combat Athletes.* Lockhart & Leith, 2016. This protocol is part of Lockhart's widely used strategies to manage water retention during fight week through herbal diuretics like dandelion root and uva ursi.

Post-Weigh-in Recovery

After successfully making weight, it's critical to rehydrate and restore electrolytes and energy. Here's a recovery plan:

- Sip on recovery shakes containing sodium, potassium, essential amino acids (EAAs), and carbohydrates. This helps to replenish electrolytes and rehydrate the body.
- Start with smaller shakes and gradually increase intake. For example, after a moderate weight cut (around 5lbs), begin with a lower sodium and potassium dose, then increase with each shake over short intervals (every 10-15 minutes).
- Eat easily digestible foods rich in sodium and potassium, such as white rice, potatoes, coconut water, or even an organic chicken noodle soup.
- Include lean proteins like boiled chicken, fish, or lean beef to support muscle recovery.
- Take digestive enzymes with meals to improve nutrient absorption.
- Stick to foods you ate during training camp to avoid adverse reactions before your fight.

Fight Day

On fight day, eat a balanced meal three to four hours before the bout to allow for proper digestion. Stay hydrated throughout the day but avoid overeating or drinking too much water too close to the fight.

The Risks of Cutting Too Much Weight

While methods like sauna suits, steam rooms, and hot bath soaks can help shed the last few pounds, they should be used sparingly and with caution. Excessive water loss can lead to dehydration, muscle cramps, and fatigue, all of which directly impact your performance on fight night. Even with 24 hours to rehydrate, your body might not fully recover, leaving you more vulnerable to damage and diminishing your stamina when it matters most.

Beyond performance, cutting too much weight can weaken your body's overall resilience. You may feel slower, out of breath, and less powerful, but even worse, your ability to absorb punches, known as "punch resistance," can drop dramatically.

Signs of Dehydration:

- Increased heart rate
- Low energy
- Dark urine

If you notice these symptoms during your cut, it's critical to rehydrate immediately and restore electrolytes. In a sport where toughness is praised, ignoring these signs can lead to serious consequences.

Always monitor your hydration levels, and consult a professional if you're unsure about any part of your cut. Taking shortcuts to hit a number on the scale isn't worth sacrificing your performance, or your safety.

I learned this the hard way. I fought at 147 pounds for most of my pro career and was determined to stay there no matter what. But by the time I fought respected welterweight contender Abel Ramos on a Premier Boxing Champions (PBC) event, live on FOX, I had clearly outgrown the weight class. In the days leading up to the weigh-in, especially the night before and the morning of, I was draining my body to hit 147. I was soaking in a hot tub, wrapped in layers, sweating it out, doing whatever it took to make weight. I was late to the weigh-ins because of it, but I made the number. I hit the target. But at what cost? I felt weakened by fight night.

Still, I had the win in mind. I trained ruthlessly in camp, and was able to dominate most of the fight with sheer punch output. But the effects of the weight cut were undeniable. In the final moments of the last round, literally with just one second left on the clock, I got caught. I stood back up on my feet, but completely fatigued. The referee waved it off, even though the final bell had technically already sounded. The result stood. That brutal cut had cost me. Thereafter, I moved up to the 154 pounds division and the difference was night and day. I felt stronger, more hydrated, and back to my true form.

Conclusion

By following a smart, scientifically informed weight-cutting plan, you can achieve your weight goals without compromising your performance. Remember, the goal goes beyond making weight; it's to enter the ring in peak condition, ready to perform at your best. Approach extreme weight cuts carefully, and consult a nutritionist or health professional for personalized advice, especially when using diuretics or water-cutting methods.

Chapter 40
The Ultimate Recovery Guide for Boxers

Recovery is the foundation of physical capacity. In the high-stakes world of boxing, every punch, every round, and every grueling training session takes a toll on your body. To stay at your best and extend your career, recovery is a must. It's the motor that drives your progress and sustains your ability to compete at a high level. This chapter explores the most effective recovery methods, focusing on practices that will help you bounce back stronger and faster. Among these methods, sleep stands out as the most powerful tool for optimal recovery and maintaining top form.

Recovery: Hard Work + Rest = Results

Boxing is about pushing your body to its limits, but success comes not simply from hard work, but from how well you recover. The phrase "no days off" might sound appealing, but without proper recovery, it's impossible to perform at your best.

For real progress, the effort must be hard and intentional. Just going through the motions won't yield significant results, even with rest. True growth happens when intense training is followed by adequate recovery. Push too hard without rest, and the result is fatigue, burnout, and injury...not progress. A 2019 study in the *Journal of Strength and Conditioning Research* found that inadequate recovery between training sessions leads to decreased performance and a higher risk of injury in combat athletes.

If you've been training hard but start feeling stale, flat, or sluggish during your sessions, don't ignore it. Those are signals that your body needs recovery. Taking 2–3 days for active recovery or complete rest can help you break through a plateau.

This window allows something called *super-compensation* to occur, where your body rebounds stronger than before, essentially giving you a supercharge of gains. This effect is most noticeable when your nutrition is also dialed in, fueling your body with clean, high-quality foods and avoiding things that impair recovery like drugs, alcohol, or junk food. Many fighters notice that after proper rest, they return sharper, faster, and more powerful.

Signs of overtraining include:

- Sleepiness or irritability
- Elevated heart rate
- Trouble sleeping
- Slower reaction times

These signs tell you it's time to dial up recovery. Effective recovery allows your body and mind to rebuild and come back stronger.

Physical methods matter, but so does the mental reset. After a fight or intense training cycle, it's important to detach from "fight mode". Take time to do things unrelated to boxing. Spend time with family, go out in nature, or dive into a hobby. Your nervous system needs space to breathe. This type of detachment isn't a weakness. It's part of coming back sharper.

Why Sleep is King

Sleep is the most powerful form of recovery. While athletes may spend hours in the gym refining their technique and strength, without proper sleep, the benefits of that hard work are limited.

During sleep, your body goes into full recovery mode, repairing the micro-tears in your muscles and releasing growth hormones like human growth hormone (HGH), which plays a critical role in rebuilding tissues. Not getting enough sleep slows this process down, leaving you vulnerable to fatigue and injury.

A 2011 study in *Sleep* showed that athletes who increased their sleep (specifically to around nine to 10 hours) saw measurable improvements in performance, including faster sprint times, better accuracy, and improved overall well-being.[53]

How to Maximize Sleep for Recovery

Here are some proven strategies to improve your sleep and accelerate your recovery:

Get 8 to 10 hours of sleep: Elite athletes often need more sleep than the average person. Floyd Mayweather, known for his sharpness in the ring, has been reported to sleep up to 10 hours a night during training.

Create a sleep-conducive environment: Keep your bedroom cool, dark, and quiet. A room temperature of 60-67°F is ideal for sleep.

Limit electronics: Avoid screens at least an hour before bed. The blue light from phones and computers disrupts your natural sleep cycle.

Establish a routine: Going to bed and waking up at the same time every day helps regulate your internal clock, making it easier to fall asleep and wake up refreshed.

Relaxation techniques: Wind down before bed with deep breathing, meditation, or reading. This helps your mind relax and prepares you for deep, restorative sleep.

Naps: A Secret Weapon

Naps can also play a key role in recovery, especially between training sessions. A short nap (20-30 minutes) is enough to boost alertness and performance without impacting your nighttime sleep. A 2007 study in the *Journal of Sports Sciences* found that even brief naps improved sprint performance and mental sharpness in athletes.[54]

---

[53] Mah, C. D., Mah, K. E., Kezirian, E. J., & Dement, W. C. (2011). "The Effects of Sleep Extension on the Athletic Performance of Collegiate Basketball Players." Sleep, 34(7), 943-950.

[54] Waterhouse, J., Atkinson, G., Edwards, B., & Reilly, T. (2007). "The role of a short post-lunch nap in improving cognitive, motor, and sprint performance in participants with partial sleep deprivation." Journal of Sports Sciences, 25(14), 1557-1566.

The Power of Saunas in Recovery

Another often overlooked but highly effective recovery tool is the sauna. Beyond just relaxation, saunas offer numerous physiological benefits that can enhance recovery for boxers.

When you sit in a sauna, your body is exposed to heat that triggers the production of heat shock proteins (HSPs), which aid in muscle repair. These proteins stabilize and refold damaged muscle fibers, helping your body recover faster after intense sessions. Saunas also boost circulation, delivering more oxygen and nutrients to your muscles.

For optimal benefits, saunas should be used at temperatures between 150-180°F (65-82°C) for 15-30 minutes per session. Beginners should start at lower temperatures and gradually build up their tolerance. Regular sauna use (two or three times per week) can significantly reduce soreness, promote faster recovery, and even improve endurance. A study in the *Journal of Science and Medicine in Sport* found that post-exercise sauna sessions improved cardiovascular endurance in athletes.[55]

How to Include Saunas into Your Routine

Post-workout recovery: Spend 15-20 minutes in a sauna after tough training sessions to relax muscles and promote recovery.

Consistency: Aim to use the sauna a couple of times a week for maximum benefits.

Hydration: Be sure to stay hydrated before and after sauna sessions. Intense sweating can lead to dehydration, which hinders recovery.

Boxers like Wladimir Klitschko have been known to incorporate regular sauna sessions into their training routines to stay at peak condition. Along with saunas, steam rooms, hot baths, and

---

[55] Stanley, J., Halliday, A., D'Auria, S., Buchheit, M., & Leicht, A. S. (2015). "Effect of sauna-based heat acclimation on plasma volume and heart rate variability." Journal of Science and Medicine in Sport, 18(1), 45-51.

infrared saunas provide similar heat therapy benefits and can be more accessible depending on your setup.

Cold Therapy: Ice Baths and Cryotherapy

Cold therapy is a highly effective way to speed up recovery, especially when it comes to reducing muscle soreness and inflammation after tough training sessions. Whether it's ice baths, cold plunges, or cryotherapy, exposing your body to cold temperatures post-workout helps reduce muscle damage and accelerate your recovery.

What Cold Therapy Does for You

Reduces soreness: After a grueling session, cold therapy helps flush out waste products like lactic acid, minimizes swelling, and reduces muscle soreness.

Boosts mental toughness: Enduring the shock of cold builds your mental resilience, which will carry over into your performance in the ring.

When Should a Boxer Use Cold Therapy?

The timing of cold therapy depends on your goal.

Fast Recovery: If your focus is on faster recovery after sparring, hard conditioning, or long pad/bag sessions, an ice bath immediately after training (10-15 minutes at 50-59°F/ 10-15°C) is ideal.

Muscle Growth: If your goal is muscle growth and strength gains, avoid ice baths right after lifting. Cold therapy reduces inflammation, which is necessary for muscle repair and growth. Instead, wait 24-48 hours before using cold therapy.

Alertness: Cold exposure before training can help with alertness and focus. A short cold shower or quick cold plunge can wake you up and prime your nervous system, which may help with explosiveness and reaction time.

Contrast Therapy: Hot–Cold Alternation

One of the most effective recovery methods for boxers is contrast therapy, which is alternating between hot and cold treatments. The rapid shift in temperature causes your blood vessels to expand and contract, pumping fresh, oxygen-rich blood into your muscles while flushing out waste products. This accelerates recovery, reduces soreness, and helps restore mobility after tough sessions.

Contrast therapy can be done with simple tools: a hot shower followed by a cold one, or alternating between a sauna and an ice bath. A common approach is 3–4 minutes of heat followed by 1–2 minutes of cold, repeated for 3–4 cycles. Fighters often find that contrast therapy not only speeds up physical recovery but also leaves them feeling recharged mentally, ready for the next day's grind.

Active Recovery: Movement Matters

While rest is key, engaging in active recovery can also help your body heal. Light activities such as swimming, cycling, or yoga help maintain blood flow to muscles, reduce stiffness, and promote healing. Active recovery between intense sessions helps maintain flexibility and prevents injury.

Additional recovery techniques like massage therapy, foam rolling, and compression therapy (from standard compression sleeves to more advanced pneumatic systems) can further enhance your recovery routine by relieving muscle tension, reducing soreness, and improving circulation. Techniques like Hyperbaric Oxygen Therapy (HBOT) are also used by some athletes to speed up healing and reduce inflammation, particularly after injuries. HBOT involves breathing pure oxygen in a pressurized chamber, which increases oxygen delivery to tissues and promotes recovery. These chambers are available at specialized medical facilities, sports recovery centers, and some high-end gyms.

Nutrition and Stretching

Although we have focused here on other important recovery methods, nutrition also plays a critical role in fueling muscle repair and replenishing energy stores (see Chapter 37), while stretching is another key component of recovery, helping to maintain flexibility, prevent injury, and reduce muscle tightness (see Chapter 35).

Wrapping It Up: Why Recovery Matters

In boxing, hard training is just part of the equation. How well you recover determines whether you continue progressing or start burning out. Alongside core practices like quality sleep, nutrition, and cold therapy, incorporating saunas and staying active on recovery days are vital for keeping your body in top condition.

Supplementary methods such as massage therapy, cupping, acupuncture, foam rolling, and compression therapy can further improve recovery, helping to relieve muscle tension and boost circulation.

Even more advanced options, like Hyperbaric Oxygen Therapy (HBOT), can accelerate healing when dealing with injuries. Recovery isn't just about repairing your body, it refreshes your mind, keeping you ready for whatever comes next.

Make recovery an essential part of your routine, and you'll be better prepared to go the distance, both in the ring and throughout your career. Remember: **Hard Work + Rest = Results.**

Round 8: Your Team

Chapter 41
Finding the Right Gym: Success Leaves Clues

"Behind every champion is a team that prepared him to become that champion." [56]
—Anderson Silva

Walking into a boxing gym for the first time can be an exciting and sometimes overwhelming experience. The energy, the sound of gloves hitting heavy bags, and the rhythm of jump ropes cutting through the air, it all sets the tone for the journey ahead. But not all gyms are the same, and finding the right one depends on your goals.

Are You Here to Fight or Get Fit?

Before choosing a gym, be clear about what you're looking for. Do you want to compete, spar, and develop real fight skills? Or is your goal to get in great shape while learning the fundamentals of boxing?

If You Want to Compete: Look for a gym with active fighters, experienced coaches, and a competitive atmosphere. A strong gym culture breeds strong fighters, so choose a place where the training is structured and the intensity is real.

If You're Training for Fitness: A boxing-based fitness gym might be a better fit. These gyms focus on conditioning, pad work, and boxing fundamentals without the full-contact intensity of a fight gym. You'll still get all the benefits of boxing training: explosiveness, agility, endurance, without needing to step into the ring.

---

[56] Silva, Anderson. Commonly attributed quote reflecting his views on teamwork and preparation. Anderson Silva is a former UFC Middleweight Champion, widely regarded as one of the greatest strikers in MMA history.

The Culture of a Gym Matters

Regardless of your goals, the gym's atmosphere should push you toward self-improvement. Some gyms focus purely on competition, while others cater to both fighters and general fitness enthusiasts. A great gym, whether competitive or fitness-based, will have coaches who care, a structured program, and an environment where people push each other to be better.

Finding the Right Fit

Before committing to a gym, try out a few. Observe how the classes or training sessions are run. Are the coaches engaged? Are members progressing? Whether you're training to fight or just to get in shape, the right gym will keep you motivated and excited to train.

That said, you don't have to be brought up in a famous or elite-level gym to become great. What matters most is the energy, hunger, and dedication of the people around you, and your own obsession to grow. A small gym with a few committed people can produce killers. Desire and discipline can outshine reputation any day of the week.

Coaches: The Architects of Champions

Finding the right coach

A great coach cannot be someone who simply holds mitts or shouts instructions. They shape your development, refine your technique, and guide your evolution as a fighter. The right coach understands your style, helps you build upon your strengths, and corrects weaknesses without forcing you into a mold that doesn't fit.

So how do you find the right one? Start by looking at their track record. Have they worked with fighters at your level or beyond? Do they understand your goals and how to get you there?

Compatibility is key. Not only in terms of personality, but in their ability to communicate in a way that resonates with you.

It's also important to observe their approach in the gym. Are they engaged with their fighters, making adjustments and giving direct feedback? Or do they seem distracted, recycling the same drills without much thought? The best coaches are fully invested in your growth, doing more than holding pads, they are teaching you how to think, react, and adapt in the ring.

The best coaches don't force a one-size-fits-all approach. They recognize that every fighter is different, with unique attributes, strengths, and instincts. They don't try to make a slick counterpuncher fight like a relentless pressure fighter, nor do they try to force a knockout artist into a defensive, point-scoring style. Instead, they work with what you bring to the table, developing your natural abilities while helping you build well-rounded skills.

At the same time, a great coach is more than just a coach. They are a teacher, strategist, and sometimes even a mentor. They help you understand the "why" behind everything you do, giving you the tools to problem-solve in real fights. A great coach doesn't just tell you what to do, they make sure you understand how to make adjustments in real-time, when it matters most.

If you're unsure about a coach, don't be afraid to test the waters. Train with different coaches, spar under their guidance, and see how their instruction impacts your performance. Some coaches work best with a particular type of fighter, while others have a broader range of expertise. Finding the right fit takes time, and you shouldn't feel locked in if something isn't working. Boxing is about evolution, and the best coaches are those who help you grow.

And just like a great fighter is always learning, a great coach never stops studying the game, sharpening their craft, and seeking new ways to bring out the best in their fighters. The sport of boxing is constantly evolving, and the best coaches stay ahead by keeping their minds open, analyzing fights, studying techniques, and learning from every fighter they work with.

They understand that to truly elevate their fighters, they must continuously elevate themselves.

In the end, a great coach is not simply someone with experience, they're someone who helps you become the best version of yourself in the ring.

Mentors: The Shortcut to Boxing Wisdom

Finding the right mentor is key to achieving your boxing goals. A good mentor provides guidance, knowledge, and the motivation needed to navigate the challenges on your path to success. Whether they're a coach or an experienced boxer, a mentor who has walked the road you're on can offer insights that can transform your journey.

A mentor is someone with the knowledge and experience you need, someone who has already been where you are trying to go. Not all mentors have been world champions themselves, but their experience and understanding of the sport are instrumental to reaching the highest levels.

Don't hesitate to seek out these mentors. Ask questions, absorb their advice, and remain open to learning. The lessons they share could be the turning point in your boxing career. I've had the privilege of learning from some of the best. Jesse Reid, a world-class coach with 29 world champions to his name, shared invaluable wisdom that shaped my approach in and out of the ring. Roy Jones Jr., one of the greatest boxers of all time, guided me through my debut in the junior middleweight division (also known as light middleweight and super welterweight, the category has a maximum weight limit of 154 lbs), expanding my understanding of the sport and introducing me to strategies and techniques I hadn't known existed.

In addition to these well-known figures, I've learned from many other coaches. Each brought their own unique perspective, contributing to my growth. From these mentors, I've gained the knowledge that I'm now passing on to you in this book.

The right mentor doesn't just offer advice; they light the way, helping you avoid pitfalls and seize opportunities. The truth is, everyone has something to teach if you're willing to listen. This openness to learning from anyone, regardless of their experience, will set you apart.

And when the moment comes in the ring, having a great coach or mentor in your corner is like having an eagle by your side. With their sharp, experienced eyes, they can see things you can't: spotting openings, reading your opponent, and guiding you with the wisdom only years in the sport can bring. Giving you the perspective and advantage you need to strike when it matters most.

I remember fighting a rugged, late-notice opponent from Tijuana, Mexico, named Victor Fonseca. He was strong, aggressive, and hit like a truck. Every shot he threw had weight behind it. I had hit him with some of the hardest counterpunches and body shots I could throw, and he just kept coming. He absorbed everything I threw with a granite chin and kept marching forward with heavy pressure and punishing shots of his own. The fight turned into a war of attrition. I began to tire from trying to take him out with pure force, and the way he kept walking through my best punches started to wear me down.

In the corner before the final round, my coach at the time, Michael Nowling, gave me a simple but crucial piece of advice: "Relax your punches and think speed. Stop trying to knock him out, just let your hands go." That one line shifted everything. I let go of trying to load up and instead focused on speed, timing, and staying loose. In that final round, I finally broke through, caught him clean, wobbled him, and closed the show.

What most people don't know is that I went into that fight with a broken nose, suffered just days before in sparring. I refused to cancel, I wasn't about to miss a shot to throw down in Vegas. I tell this story because it's a reminder: sometimes, the right words from your corner can change the entire outcome of a fight.

The Dream Team: Strength in Numbers

When the bell rings, it's just you and your opponent in the ring. But getting to that moment? That's a team effort. No boxer climbs to the top alone, it takes a dedicated group of people all working together to help you succeed.

Your team is like your secret weapon. Coaches fine-tune your technique and strategy, nutritionists make sure you're fueling right, and trainers push your physical limits. Physiotherapists help you recover and stay injury-free, while strength coaches build the endurance and power you need to go the distance.

Some boxers even work with mental coaches to keep their eyes on the prize when the pressure's on. And, of course, sparring partners are there to give you that real fight feel before the main event.

A well-functioning team doesn't just consist of great individuals; it thrives on collaboration. Although egos can sometimes get in the way, true greatness happens when there is unity among the coaches. When they're all aligned with the same vision, their collective efforts form a powerful mastermind alliance. This synergy elevates the fighter and the entire team, pushing everyone to new levels of success.

With that being said, it's not simply about having a team, it's about how seamlessly they work together. When communication flows and everyone contributes toward the same goal, you create a strong foundation that allows you to focus on what you do best. As the saying goes, *"Teamwork makes the dream work."* Every role is important, and together, they give you the advantage you need.

When you finally step into that ring, you're not alone. Every punch, every move, every victory? It's backed by the hours of work your team put in with you. And that's the beauty of boxing. Even though you fight alone, success is always a shared effort.

But What If You Don't Have a Full Team?

Although having a full team is ideal, what if you don't have access to all that support? It's not about the resources you have, but how resourceful you can be. Not every boxer has access to state-of-the-art facilities and expert coaches, yet many have gone on to become world champions. Some fighters come from places where boxing knowledge and gyms are limited. So, if you're in that situation, don't sweat it, that's why you've got this book! You can still sharpen your skills by breaking down fight footage, shadowboxing with intent, and applying the principles in this guide. World-class fighters have come from nothing but grit, hunger, and a willingness to learn.

When access is limited, it's all about creativity and determination. You may need to travel outside of your comfort zone to find better training, new sparring partners, or if need be, more experienced coaches. Pushing yourself by sparring with different fighters, facing new challenges, and experiencing those intense emotions will help you grow as a boxer. The reality is, most opportunities lie outside of your comfort zone, and that's where real growth happens. Many fighters have found success by seeking out these new experiences, and so can you.

Even if you're from a place with a smaller boxing community or fewer options, success is still within your reach. Use what's available, challenge yourself, and don't be afraid to venture into unfamiliar territory. It's through those uncomfortable situations where you'll discover your true potential.

Chapter 42
Nature vs Nurture: The Great Debate, Settled

No one is born with perfect footwork, flawless timing, or an endless gas tank. Every fighter starts awkward, missing shots and making mistakes. What separates the great from the rest isn't talent, it's what comes next.

People love the idea of talent because it gives them an excuse. If greatness is something you're born with, they don't have to try their best. But that's a lie we tell ourselves to justify mediocrity.

Talent may give someone an early advantage, but it's the relentless work, persistence through failure, and the discipline to learn and improve that truly builds skill. Greatness isn't something you're born with, it's something you earn through hours of dedication.

Look at the best fighters in history: They also happen to be the hardest workers. That's not a coincidence. The ones who rise to the top aren't just born with talent; they outwork everyone to get there. But it's not limited to working the hardest, it's about working the smartest. Knowing how to train, what to prioritize, and when to recover separates the truly elite from those who burn out or plateau.

Take Roy Jones Jr., whose lightning-fast speed and incredible agility shook up the boxing world. While these natural gifts were undeniable, it was the countless hours in the gym that transformed them into world-class skills. Floyd Mayweather Jr.'s defensive brilliance didn't come from talent alone. His obsessive attention to detail and endless practice allowed him to master the sport. Mike Tyson's legendary power was developed through disciplined, repetitive training, making him one of the most feared fighters in history.

I've seen this play out in my own journey. When I first stepped into a competitive boxing gym, I wasn't the most talented fighter in the room. There were guys with more experience, sharper skills, and a natural edge. But I kept showing up. Day after day, I put in the work, staying consistent and hungry. Over time, I caught up. And eventually, I surpassed them. It wasn't talent that got me there, it was consistency, discipline, and the willingness to outwork everyone else in the room.

In the end, it's not about who starts with the most talent. It's about who can turn potential into mastery through consistent effort, persistence, and a refusal to quit.

The Daily Grind: What Separates the Best

"I'm not here to be average, I'm here to be the best." [57]

Boxing is more than just a sport. It's a lifestyle, demanding discipline and an unbreakable commitment to improvement. While talent may set the stage, what truly separates the elite is their ability to show up, day after day, and work their craft. In the ring, it's more than the ability to throw and dodge a punch that matters. It's the ability to do it over and over again, better each time.

To achieve greatness, or even just to reach your personal best, you must develop an unwavering routine. It's the decision to train, work on your technique, and push through when your body or mind wants to quit, that's what fuels progress and separates the elite from everyone else.

You don't rise from the pack by showing up when it's convenient. You rise by showing up when it's uncomfortable, when it's hard, and when no one is watching.

It's more than just talent, and it's not about how good you are on your best day. It's about how good you can be on your worst day, and whether you can stay focused through pain, exhaustion, or setbacks. Consistent effort builds skill and resilience, layer by

---

[57] Common motivational quote; widely circulated in athletic and self-development contexts without verifiable attribution..

layer, over time. The greatest boxers aren't obsessed with perfection in one moment, they're committed to the daily grind that leads to mastery.

Obsession: The Fuel for Excellence

"Be more than motivated...become literally obsessed...people think you're nuts."[58]—David Goggins

Obsession is more than a trait. It's a necessity for those striving to be the best. It drives the relentless pursuit of improvement, pushing athletes to reach new heights, both physically and mentally. It fuels a burning desire beyond winning, but to master the sport, achieve excellence, and leave a lasting legacy. It goes beyond money, fame, or titles. It's about pushing the boundaries of what's possible and constantly seeking improvement.

This obsession reveals itself in a boxer's daily routine. The best fighters train relentlessly, always striving to perfect their technique, improve their physical fitness, and build their mental toughness. They don't see limits; they only see challenges to overcome. And while many might view this intensity as extreme, it's the very trait that defines the most iconic fighters in history.

The Importance of Habits and The Compound Effect

"Champions aren't made in the ring, they are merely recognized there. What you cheat on in the early light of morning will show up in the ring under the bright lights." [59] —Joe Frazier

---

[58] David Goggins, *Can't Hurt Me: Master Your Mind and Defy the Odds* (Lioncrest Publishing, 2018), Chapter 5.

[59] Joe Frazier, as quoted in *Box Like the Pros* by Joe Frazier and William Dettloff (New York: HarperCollins, 2005), 4.

You might look at a highly skilled fighter and wonder if you could ever reach that level. The truth is, it's simply a matter of time and dedication to the craft compounded over weeks, months, and years. The fighter you see didn't become great overnight. It's the result of countless hours spent in the gym, perfecting their craft, day after day. This same principle works for you. The more you commit to daily improvement, the more you will grow as a fighter. The key is to focus on the process, not the result. Each day spent training, even when progress feels slow, is a necessary part of the journey. Sacrifice is your companion on this path, and it will bring you closer to success.

As you continue to train, you will gradually get better and better, often without even realizing it. This transformation happens so subtly that you might not notice the progress day-to-day, but over time, the small improvements compound into massive gains. Each punch, each drill, each conditioning session adds up, and one day you'll look back and see how far you've come. The compound effect means that the accumulation of small, consistent actions leads to significant improvements in your overall performance.

Habits play a major role in achieving greatness. Good ones run like a well-oiled machine, moving you toward your goals. Bad ones are sand in the gears, creating friction and slowing everything down. To keep progressing without interruption, it's important to develop positive habits and clear out the negative ones that create resistance.

> *"We are what we repeatedly do. Excellence,*
> *then, is not an act, but a habit."* [60]
> —Will Durant, summarizing Aristotle

However, it's important to recognize that the compound effect can also work against you. Consistently engaging in bad habits can lead to negative outcomes in the ring. Therefore, it's crucial to consistently engage in positive habits and behaviors. By doing

---

[60] Durant, Will. "The Story of Philosophy" (New York: Simon & Schuster, 1926), summarizing Aristotle's "Nicomachean Ethics," Book II. While commonly attributed directly to Aristotle, this phrasing is Durant's interpretation of Aristotelian philosophy.

this, you create a momentum that drives continuous improvement over time.

Mastery: The Ultimate Goal

Mastery represents the pinnacle of understanding and achievement in any field. It requires intense focus, dedication, and a level of commitment that goes beyond natural talents or abilities. Achieving this level of expertise demands deep immersion, a mindset geared toward continuous learning, and an unwavering drive to improve your knowledge and skills.

The journey to becoming an expert is built on repetition. It's not enough to practice once and move on; true excellence comes from honing your abilities through consistent practice and experimentation. Each time you train, you build muscle memory and sharpen your technique. Practice doesn't just make perfect, it leads to lasting improvement. Through steady effort, you gradually elevate your abilities until they reach expert levels.

The Theory of Addition Through Subtraction is critical in this process. Sometimes, to achieve more, you need to focus on less. This means eliminating distractions, bad habits, and anything that doesn't contribute to your goals. By removing negative influences, whether it's unhealthy foods, pessimistic friends, or unnecessary distractions, you create space for higher-quality practice, recovery, and focus. This concept is key to excelling in your craft, as it helps you prioritize what truly matters and accelerates your progress.

Finding a mentor can also speed up your journey. A mentor offers valuable feedback, helps you avoid common pitfalls, and provides guidance on how to achieve long-term success. With their support, combined with your unwavering dedication, the path to excellence becomes much clearer.

Consistency in Action

Success isn't the result of one grand effort, but the accumulation of daily actions. Dedication, positive habits, and the compound effect are powerful tools, but they all rely on one thing, consistency. Every small action counts, and over time, these actions build on each other to create a champion.

The true mark of a champion isn't just talent or hard work, it's the ability to show up every day, put in the work, and never let up. That's what separates the great from the good. Talent may start the race, but obsession, discipline, and unbreakable consistency finish it. That's the line that separates the great from the good, and it's the line legends cross.

Beyond the Gym: Combining Cross-Training and Creative Insight in Boxing

Getting Started

Boxing training is intense, hours in the gym, working on technique, strength, conditioning, and cardio. But what if you could add something different to push your performance even further? Cross-training isn't about training more, it's about expanding your approach to it. By stepping outside of the usual routine and incorporating diverse activities, you can sharpen your skills, boost your fitness, and uncover new ways to improve your game. This type of creative, well-rounded training helps you break through plateaus and unlock strengths you didn't even know you had. Cross-training pushes you beyond the limits of traditional training, making you a more adaptable and dynamic athlete by changing how you move, think, and respond.

How Athletes Benefit from Cross-Training

Many elite fighters have turned to cross-training, integrating other sports and activities to improve their boxing:

Sergio Martinez and Soccer: Martinez's background in soccer gave him powerful lower-body conditioning and exceptional stamina. His time on the field sharpened his footwork and endurance, allowing him to glide effortlessly in the ring and maintain his energy deep into fights.

Manny Pacquiao and Basketball: Pacquiao, an avid basketball player, has long enjoyed the sport's fast pace and constant movement. This activity naturally kept him light on his feet and quick in the ring, with many skills from the court carrying over to his boxing.

Evander Holyfield and Ballet: Ballet provided Holyfield with remarkable balance and coordination. The precision required in ballet helped him improve his movement in the ring, allowing him to control space more effectively and maintain stability during exchanges.

Vasiliy Lomachenko and Ukrainian Dance: Lomachenko's father introduced him to traditional Ukrainian dance as part of his training. This form of dance focused on rhythm, coordination, and intricate footwork, giving him exceptional fluidity and control. Lomachenko's ability to pivot, shift angles, and evade punches stems from the skills he developed through dance.

Cross-training brings variety to your training regimen, targeting different physical attributes and helping you develop a more complete set of skills. By expanding beyond boxing-specific drills, you can become a more versatile athlete, ready for any challenge.

What is Creative Insight?

Creative insight is about finding solutions or techniques that go beyond conventional training. For boxers, it often involves drawing from different experiences or unusual disciplines to heighten performance and bring a fresh perspective to their craft.

Why Thinking Creatively Matters in Boxing

Thinking outside the box allows you to tap into strategies or techniques from unexpected places, helping you develop a unique advantage in the ring. Several top fighters have applied creative insights from other arts and sports to push their game to the next level:

Sugar Ray Robinson and Tap Dancing: Sugar Ray Robinson turned to tap dancing to improve his movement in the ring. The rhythm and timing developed through tap allowed him to move with grace and agility, often leaving opponents swinging at air.

Joe Calzaghe and Music: Joe Calzaghe's father had him train in sync with music, using beats to help him perfect his timing and coordination. This rhythm-based training contributed to Calzaghe's relentless pace in the ring, overwhelming his opponents with continuous, well-timed combinations.

Roy Jones Jr. and Roosters: Jones found inspiration in nature, particularly in observing how roosters fought. He noted how they used quick, sudden attacks and unpredictable angles, and he applied these tactics to his boxing style. His dynamic movements often left opponents mesmerized.

Bruce Lee and Fencing: Bruce Lee revolutionized martial arts by integrating principles from fencing, such as quick, precise footwork and distance control. These techniques made him elusive in combat, allowing him to maintain control while staying one step ahead of his opponents.

Lennox Lewis and Chess: Lennox Lewis's interest in chess significantly influenced his strategic thinking in the ring. Chess develops patience, foresight, and the ability to anticipate an opponent's moves, skills that Lewis used to outthink and outmaneuver his rivals.

Salsa Dancing and Footwork: Later in my career, I took up salsa dancing to improve my footwork, rhythm, and balance. The fast-paced footwork and constant shifts in direction that salsa demands helped me develop quicker, more fluid movements. This translated directly into my boxing, allowing me to pivot and adjust angles with more ease and confidence.

These creative insights show how boxing can be evolved through unconventional methods, helping you develop new skills and approaches that are difficult for opponents to anticipate.

Bringing It All Together

Blending cross-training with outside-the-box thinking helps you develop into a well-rounded, adaptive, and mentally sharp fighter. Like the athletes who found inspiration from soccer, dance, or even nature, you can integrate outside influences to enhance both your physical and mental performance. This continuous growth not only makes you a more complete fighter but also equips you to rise above the competition.

Chapter 43
The Eternal Student

*"There are no limits. There are only plateaus, and
you must not stay there. You must go beyond them."* [61]
—Bruce Lee

As you reach the final pages of this book, one truth stands above all: no matter how far you rise in boxing, you must always remain a student. The greatest champions never stop learning. Whether you're a veteran or a rising star, growth in this sport is never over.

Boxing evolves constantly, with new techniques and strategies emerging. To stay ahead, keep an open mind and adapt. Complacency is the downfall of many fighters, curiosity and a hunger for knowledge will set you apart.

Adaptation keeps you dangerous. Whether refining a punch combination or developing new skills, your ability to evolve ensures longevity in the sport. Just as boxing advances, so must you.

Learn from coaches, trainers, fellow fighters, and even sports scientists. Study fights, analyze strategies, and absorb wisdom from every corner. The broader your knowledge, the more complete your skill set.

Win or lose, each fight reveals valuable insights. Celebrate what worked, but focus on where you can improve. Success confirms strengths; failure exposes weaknesses. Both fuel your growth.

Breakthroughs come from stepping outside your comfort zone. Don't be afraid to test new techniques. Innovation keeps you unpredictable and sharp.

---

[61] Lee, Bruce. Quoted in "The Art of Expressing the Human Body," ed. John R. Little (Tuttle Publishing, 1998), p. 23. Also referenced from televised interview archives.

Study the greats, but don't get stuck in tradition. Learn from history while staying ahead of modern advancements. This balance will shape your unique path to success.

The tools are in your grasp. It's up to you to apply them. The discipline, focus, and perseverance boxing instills will serve you well beyond the ring.

Now, as everything you've read comes together, remember: true mastery comes from never losing the desire to grow. Keep learning, keep pushing, and give it everything you've got. The ring is waiting. Your destiny is in your hands.

Before we part ways, I want to leave you with one last truth.

There's something I didn't know when I started writing this book, and it changed everything.

I boxed for more than 20 years, pushing through surgeries and complications no one could fully explain. During recovery from a hand surgery, while preparing for a possible return to the ring, I finally found the answer. I had unknowingly fought my entire career with Hemophilia B, a rare bleeding disorder.

It explains a lot. The bleeding. The setbacks. The risks I didn't even know I was taking. And ultimately, it is the reason I have to step away from the ring.

But the fight isn't over. The mindset, the knowledge, the lessons, they all come with me. I may not compete in the same way again, but I'll keep building. Teaching. Creating. And I'll keep fighting, just from a different corner.

I'll continue to be the eternal student I encourage you to be.

You've got the blueprint now. What you do with it... that's your fight.

www.ingramcontent.com/pod-product-compliance
Lightning Source LLC
Chambersburg PA
CBHW051505120626
46551CB00012B/784